Introduction to
THE OPERATING ROOM

Edited by

Amalia Cochran, MD, FACS, FCCM
Associate Professor of Surgery
Vice Chair of Education and Professionalism
University of Utah Department of Surgery
Salt Lake City, Utah

Ruth Braga, MSN, RN
Surgery Education Coordinator
University of Utah Department of Surgery
Salt Lake City, Utah

New York / Chicago/ San Francisco / Athens / London /
Madrid / Mexico City / Milan / New Delhi / Singapore /
Sydney / Toronto

Introduction to the Operating Room

1 2 3 4 5 6 7 8 9   DSS   21 20 19 18 17 16

ISBN 978-1-259-58728-3
MHID 1-259-58728-2

This book was set in Minion Pro by Cenveo® Publisher Services.
The editors were Brian Belval and Christie Naglieri.
The production supervisor was Richard Ruzycka.
Project Management was provided by Raghavi Khullar, Cenveo Publisher Services.
The cover designer was Dreamit, Inc.
Cover image credit: Spotmatikphoto/123RF.
The index was prepared by Robert Swanson.

Library of Congress Cataloging-in-Publication Data

Names: Cochran, Amalia, editor. | Braga, Ruth, editor.
Title: Introduction to the operating room / edited by Amalia Cochran, Ruth Braga.
Description: New York : McGraw-Hill Education, [2017] | Includes bibliographical
    references and index.
Identifiers: LCCN 2016009504| ISBN 9781259587283 (pbk.) |
    ISBN 1259587282 (pbk.)
Subjects: | MESH: Operating Rooms—organization & administration |
    Patient Care Team—organization & administration | Medical Staff,
    Hospital—psychology | Cooperative Behavior | Communication |
    Surgical Procedures, Operative
Classification: LCC RD63 | NLM WX 200 | DDC 617.9/17—dc23 LC record available at
http://lccn.loc.gov/2016009504

From Amalia:
To my Mom for teaching me how to be a teacher and for fostering my curiosity.
To Danny Custer for showing me how to be a kind, successful, and happy surgeon.
To my learners for inspiring me every time you have a "Gee Whiz!" moment.

From Ruth:
To my husband Michael, who encouraged me to go to nursing school
(despite my fear of blood) and supported me through everything that followed it.
For Brandon, Mindy, and Nick for reminding me that life is precious.
To everyone who continues to take a chance on me—thank you.

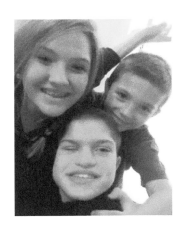

Contents

Our OR Team

Editors

Ruth Braga, MSN, RN
Department of Surgery
University of Utah
Salt Lake City, Utah
@RuthBragaMSN

Amalia Cochran, MD, FACS, FCCM
Department of Surgery
University of Utah
Salt Lake City, Utah
@AmaliaCochranMD

Contributors

Sebrena Banecker, RN, BSN, CNOR
Clinical Nurse Coordinator—
    Operating Room
Huntsman Cancer Institute
Salt Lake City, Utah

Christopher J. Behrens, MD
Department of Anesthesiology
University of Utah
Salt Lake City, Utah

Ross M. Blagg, MD
Division of Plastic Surgery
University of Utah
Salt Lake City, Utah

Marie Crandall, MD, MPH, FACS
Department of Surgery
University of Florida
Jacksonville, Florida
@vegansurgeon

Thaona D. Garber, RN
Burn Trauma Intensive Care Unit
University of Utah
Salt Lake City, Utah

Brian J. Gavitt, MD, MPH
Division of Trauma Surgery
LA County + USC Medical Center
Los Angeles, California

Elizabeth Hanes, BSN, RN
Inkslinger Communications, LLC
Houston, Texas
@EHanesRN

Cynthia Howard, RN, CNC, PhD
Vibrant Radiant Health, LLC
Santa Barbara, California
@masterwellbeing

Louise Hull, PhD
Center for Implementation Science
Kings College
London, UK

Christian Jones, MD, FACS
Division of Acute Care Surgery
Johns Hopkins University
    School of Medicine
Baltimore, Maryland
@jonesssurgery

Halle Kogan, BSN, RN, CCRN
Burn Trauma Intensive Care Unit
University of Utah
Salt Lake City, Utah

Walter Medlin, MD, FACS
Bariatric Medicine Institute
Salt Lake City, Utah
@bonuslife

Jennie O'Shea, BS, CCP
Department of Surgery
University of Utah
Salt Lake City, Utah

Karen Porter, BSN, RN
Department of Clinical Education
University of Utah
Salt Lake City, Utah

Luke V. Selby, MD
Department of Surgery
Memorial Sloan Kettering
    Cancer Center
New York, New York
Department of General Surgery
University of Colorado
Denver, Colorado
@lvselbs

Lara Senekjian, MD, MAT
Department of Surgery
University of Utah
Salt Lake City, Utah

Nick Sevdalis, PhD
Center for Implementation Science
Kings College
London, United Kingdom

Lawrence A. Shirley, MD
Division of Surgical Oncology
The Ohio State University
    College of Medicine
Columbus, Ohio
@drewshirleymd

Clive (CJ) Thirkill, MSN, CRNA
Department of Anesthesiology
University of Utah
Salt Lake City, Utah

Madeline B. Torres, MD
Department of Surgery
Penn State Hershey Medical Center
Hershey, Pennsylvania
@madelinebtorres

Diane Tyler, MSN, RN
Department of Anesthesiology
University of Utah
Salt Lake City, Utah

Thomas K. Varghese Jr., MD,
MS, FACS
Department of Surgery
University of Utah
Salt Lake City, Utah
@TomVargheseJr

Crystal D. Webb, PA-C
Department of Surgery
University of Utah
Salt Lake City, Utah

Jon Worthen, MSN, RN, CNOR
Nursing Faculty
Westminster College School of
    Nursing
Salt Lake City, Utah

Preface

Our interest in writing this book grew out of our common commitment to the OR being a "civilized" and respectful environment. We want it to be a place where learners can do so effectively, and where patients receive high quality care. In order for those things to happen, the OR needs to be a space of curiosity and questions and growth.

We also recognize that things in the OR typically occur at lightning speed, which can make it hard to have any concept of what is happening. And, of course, as a newbie to the OR, sometimes you just don't want to ask. Here's how we see the basic equation driving that behavior:

Completely foreign environment
+ Mystique of "surgical personalities" (they eat their young, right?)

+ Beehive-like activity in the OR

No WAY am I asking a question.

The reality is that no one expects you to show up in the OR on day one and know it all. And while we do hope that you'll ask questions to prevent you from making missteps, this book is also designed to help walk you through some common issues.

We can't change the nature of the work in the OR, and we're trying to change the culture of surgery for the good. What we can do right now is help manage the information flow to support you, the OR novice, and help alleviate your anxiety and normalize your experiences.

Welcome to our OR.

Pre-Op (Before the OR)

A. Know Before You Go

CHAPTER 1

The Operating Room as a Study in Cultural Anthropology

• *Amalia Cochran, MD, FACS, FCCM*

Imagine yourself dropped off on an island, or perhaps even another planet, with living beings who appear similar to humans that you know. You know little to nothing about who they are, what their lives are like, what things they do, how they do things, how they interact as a group. You may not know their language, and you definitely don't know anything about their shared traditions. You don't know their values and stories. All you know is that you are in a place with different sights, smells, sounds than anyplace you have ever been before, surrounded by other beings who seem very different from any you have experienced and who are doing things that appear to be a bit crazy and frightening.

You may have just "discovered" a previously unknown culture. Or you may be in the operating room.

*****

Are you familiar with Margaret Mead? Allow me to briefly introduce her work to you. Dr. Mead was an anthropologist largely credited with advancing the field of cultural anthropology by immersing herself with the groups she studied in Samoa and New Guinea. Cultural anthropology is distinct from other types of anthropology in that it focuses on cultural variation among humans. Because of this, cultural anthropology can provide a meaningful lens for someone new to an existing cultural environment.

Think about it ... here you are, suddenly cast into a completely unfamiliar place. When you first arrive in the OR, almost everything about it is likely to feel unnatural to you and may even be a bit horrifying; at minimum it's likely to seem weird. By coming into this space, you get the opportunity to observe firsthand the completely unique tribe of the OR on the island of surgery. Entering the OR allows you to be a participant with your presence, but you also have the opportunity to be an observer of almost everything that the tribe does while you are there. Questions you might ask include the following:

- How does the tribe work together?
- Are there any apparent rituals for the tribe?
- What patterns or symbols do you notice? Remember that language can be a symbol.
- Are there any shared myths you hear?
- How does key knowledge pass between tribe members?
- What power structures do you see among tribe members?
- What kinds of technology does the tribe have, and how do they use it?

By being in the OR, you get the chance to see firsthand how all of these things impact the island of surgery and the care of the surgical patient. **What questions does being in this new place raise for you?**

One of the challenges of being fully immersed in a strange culture or subculture is the possibility of projecting your own experiences and expectations onto the new culture. It's human nature to use what we know as our "lens" for looking at the world, and this can be particularly true when one enters an intimidating environment, as the OR often is for people. As someone new to the OR, you may not have experienced or observed all of the rituals, or may not have all of the information about them (even after reading this book). When you find yourself struggling to understand what is happening and wanting to judge it, that can be an important time to ask questions to help you gain insight from the perspective of members of the OR tribe. Remember, though, that if a situation has become life threatening it is best to hold on to your questions until the situation is resolved. However, many of us in the operating room environment truly enjoy sharing our stories and perspectives with those who are new. **What do you feel being in this new place as you watch what is happening?**

Use your experiences observing and participating in the operating room as a time and place to stay curious and to carefully observe *everything*. Consider your-self an adventurer cast into a new place, and use that to learn without assumptions or prejudice. As someone new to this place, you have the ability to perceive things that have become the norm to those of us who are part of the tribe, and sometimes they are things that we could be doing better. Sometimes if we listen carefully we can learn from you as the novice.

Welcome to our island. I hope you'll have a good stay here (Figure 1.1).

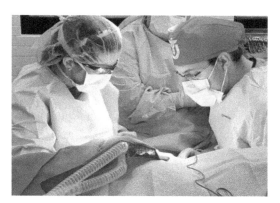

FIGURE 1.1 Whether you are new to the tribe or have been around the island, there is always some-thing to learn from one another. Watch, participate, learn, teach, and enjoy! (Photo used with permission from Ruth Braga, University of Utah.)

From Start to Finish: Understanding How We Get Here

• *Ruth Braga, MSN, RN*

It is often said that one either loves or hates the operating room (OR), with nothing in between. Some say that our roles are too dependent on others and that the OR is boring because of this. If you are preparing to shadow someone, visit as a student, select surgery as a career, or have surgery yourself, we hope that this book will provide you with enough information to have a meaningful and safe experience in the OR. If we've done our job well, it might even be fun.

To feel prepared, you need to understand the basic flow of how a patient comes to the operating room. The exact details, order, and process of the operative experience will vary by location, policy, and individual patient situation. We have tried to generalize as much as possible. If you have questions about your experience, please discuss these with your physician, instructor, or an OR staff member. Just as some of our photos are blurry (patient privacy, you know), we've tried to paint the OR experience in broad brushstrokes. Every experience is unique.

■ WHAT DO YOU KNOW ABOUT THE OPERATING ROOM?

Many people gain what knowledge they have about the OR from watching medical dramas on television. If you are someone who has relied on television depictions, let me be the first in this book to say it: that's not how things really work. Some people gain knowledge of the OR from their experience as a patient. Personal experience can be valuable but it is likely you don't remember much after rolling into the room.

To start you off on a realistic foot, we do *not* always operate in the dark (this is only done in certain cases), scrub without our masks on, or see the OR as the prime location for romance to develop (although it does happen on occasion).

On the other hand, we *do:*

- Experience drama
- Joke around with each other
- Get a little choked up from time to time (we hide it well behind our mask)
- Feel moments of high anxiety for our colleagues and patients
- Wipe sweat from, or scratch the brow of others
- Expose ourselves to dangerous situations (you won't get any closer to bodily fluids than in the OR)
- Count more often than the Count on Sesame Street
- Get a bird's eye view of the amazing things that the body is capable of

■ TEAMWORK RULES

Of the many tips and suggestions throughout this book, please remember the most important concept: it takes a team to function optimally in the OR.

Every aspect of care that we discuss involves and impacts more than one person. When everyone works together, the OR is a well-tuned symphony. We each have our solo moment(s) to be in the spotlight, but even when it is not our turn, it is impossible to provide complete care without the full dedication of each individual. When a person resists the work of others on the team, feels that they are not part of the team, or refuses to recognize the role and purpose of others, the symphony falls apart and the care and safety of the patient begin to hit out-of-tune notes.

■ WE NEED TO OPERATE

The decision perform do surgery is not always an easy or straightforward one. Surgery can be performed to diagnose, rule out, repair, prevent, start, stop, or enhance a condition. Sometimes a surgeon will not know what he or she is dealing with until they do surgery. Sometimes surgery is planned and scheduled. Sometimes, such as in a trauma situation, the decision for surgery is made in the blink of an eye. Although there are consistencies in similar operative cases, no two cases are ever alike.

■ DO YOU UNDERSTAND WHAT WILL BE DONE?

Although the patient may ask their regular physician, friends, or Google for answers about their upcoming operation, it is critical that they discuss the details with the surgeon and provide informed consent (Figure 2.1). The surgeon explains the procedure and reviews any potential side effects or problems that could occur, and what these might mean for the patient. The surgeon also will discuss alternatives to surgery with the patient (even when those alternatives aren't necessarily realistic options). This discussion occurs in the office or immediately prior to surgery. The consent is a legal document and this conversation must take place when the patient has not had any medications or is otherwise influenced—the patient

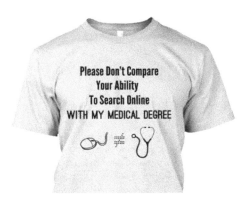

FIGURE 2.1 T-shirt designed by Ruth Braga MSN, RN. (Photo used with permission from Ruth Braga, University of Utah.)

must have "capacity" to make decisions about their care. This is a great chance to ask questions, and surgery can be declined if a patient is against it. Consent forms come with a large amount of fine print. Patient questions are welcome during a robust consent process.

■ SO YOU'RE GOING TO HAVE AN OPERATION …

Once the surgery date has been set and everything is scheduled, the patient receives very specific preparation instructions. These vary depending on the type of surgery but can include directions on eating, bathing, shaving, medications, and so forth.

One of the most inconvenient surgery preps involves cleansing of the bowels for abdominal surgery. If you are having a surgery that requires a bowel prep, you will need unrestricted access to a functioning toilet. If you question whether you truly need to choke down the unusually large prescribed amount of the cleansing agent, just remember, it is always safer to have clean bowels at the time of surgery.

Step Away from the Food and Drink

Sometimes this can be the most difficult preparation of all, especially for small children or impatient adults. Nothing should be eaten for a certain number of hours prior to surgery if the patient is going to have sedation or a general anesthetic. Make sure the patient understands when to be NPO (taking nothing by mouth). Many don't realize how significant this instruction is, but if there is anything at all in the stomach there is a chance it could inadvertently enter the esophagus or lungs. Ignoring the NPO instruction will result in postponed or cancelled surgery. If the patient is on medication, they will be given specific instructions about how and when to take those medications prior to surgery.

■ TAKE IT ALL OFF!

The day for surgery has arrived and the patient checks in. If the patient is coming from home, a family member or friend should bring them to the pre-operative

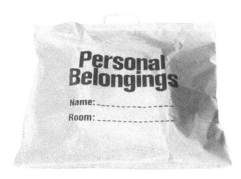

FIGURE 2.2 Leave your valuables at home—everything else goes in this bag. (Photo used with permission from Ruth Braga, University of Utah.)

area of the hospital or surgery center. Once the patient is checked in, they will be asked to change out of their street clothing into a surgical gown and tuck their hair into a shower cap-looking hat. If you think finding a hair in your food is nasty, we're pretty sure you don't want to find one in your surgical site. Don't worry—everyone who goes into the OR gets to model this look.

This is also the time for personal items to be taken off and packed away (Figure 2.2). These items can get lost or present safety hazards: fingers swell during surgery from the fluids that are given, so rings pose a threat to circulation. Your patient may be fine taking off their wedding ring and handing it to a family member for safekeeping. If they're removing eyeglasses or hearing aids, the anxiety and discomfort level significantly increases. Take extra care to help them stay comfortable, involved, and informed.

In order to instill fluids and other necessary medications, an IV must be started. A word of caution: before beginning an IV, it is a good idea to ask family members or friends if they want to stay. If so, make sure they are seated. Always make sure your patient is lying down or seated when beginning an IV. You never know how they might react to seeing an IV start or a little bit of blood. The last thing you want is for someone to pass out.

■ LET THE QUESTIONING BEGIN!

The anesthesiologist (see Chapter 4) will visit and ask about patient history, allergies, what and when the patient last ate, the procedure that is going to be done, and any conditions that might affect the ability to use anesthesia or sedation. Answering these questions honestly is imperative because the smallest detail can influence outcomes. If general anesthesia is going to be used, the anesthesiologist will assess the patient's teeth, mouth, and jaw. You'd be surprised to know how much the mouth and jaw are moved around in order to get that breathing tube in place! If this is going to be a problem for the patient, now is the time for them to speak up.

The circulator (a registered nurse who will be in the OR; see Chapter 4) will see the patient and ask questions regarding allergies, NPO status, and procedure. They will review the consent form and make sure all of the information matches. The nurse will ask the patient if they have any metal in their body because this

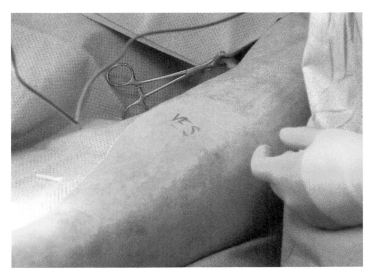

FIGURE 2.3 A simple "yes" is all you need. The marking must show even after the patient's skin has been prepped. (Photo used with permission from Ruth Braga, University of Utah.)

can influence how electrocautery is handled during surgery (see Chapter 10). Information about any prior surgeries or injuries will help to ensure the patient is positioned in the safest and most comfortable way.

The surgeon or surgeons (see Chapter 4) will then come to see the patient and once again may ask many of the same questions. They may do a physical exam and ask how the prep (if any) went. The patient may ask any other questions that have come up since they last met. If the surgery is taking place in a teaching hospital, residents (see Chapter 4) and medical students (see Chapter 4) may ask these questions in addition to the surgeon. The surgeon will mark the patient where they are going to be operated on and ask the patient to confirm it (Figure 2.3). Even when it is obvious, we want to make sure everyone understands exactly what will be done.

Why Do You Ask?

While our questions may be annoying, each person who talks to the patient has a different reason for asking. Sometimes one person hears or notices something that was previously missed. It may seem silly, but I have seen a patient say "left" while pointing to the "right," or a surgeon write something on the consent form that the patient was unaware of. Everyone (especially the patient) appreciates it when we notice a discrepancy before getting started. This is teamwork in action.

■ TIME TO ROLL

When everything checks out, all questions have been answered, and the OR is ready, the patient will say goodbye to their family member or friend and be taken

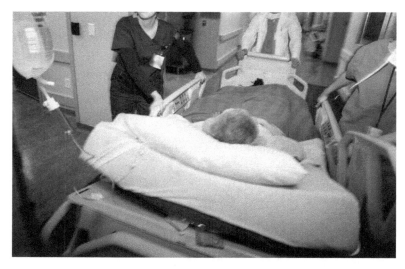

FIGURE 2.4 After saying goodbyes, the patient is rolled down the hallway to the OR. (Photo used with permission from Charlie Ehlert, University of Utah.)

to the operating room. Visitors will go to the waiting room where the surgeon can find and talk to them when the procedure is completed.

Even if the patient is able to walk, they will be placed on a bed or stretcher (Figure 2.4). Although this may seem awkward, it is safer to be lying down entering the OR. The anesthesiologist has started fluids and often has given some relaxing medication in the IV. Reassure the patient and let them know they're going to get excellent care. Offer them the best part of the operating room: warm blankets.

■ IT'S FREEZING IN HERE

As the patient rolls through the door, the OR can be an intimidating site (Figure 2.5). Multiple machines are running, screens may be lit up, everyone is masked with matching scrubs and puffy hats on their heads, surgical instruments are open or being opened, multiple individuals are moving about, and many conversations may be going on. Although this might be just another day at work for staff, keep in mind that it is an unsettling sight for the patient. All attention should focus on the patient's comfort and safety. We try to keep things calm by minimizing conversation, turning off any music that may have been playing, keeping everyone focused on the patient, and being ready to provide a helping hand to anesthesia if needed when the patient comes into the room.

The patient needs to be moved from the stretcher to the OR bed (sometimes referred to as the OR table), always under anesthesia's guidance, so they can prepare the patient to go to sleep. To do this, the stretcher that the patient was rolled into the room on is pulled up right next to the OR bed as tightly as possible.

If the patient is unconscious or otherwise unable to move, the OR staff will need to assist. Aside from the scrub technician (usually setting up instruments

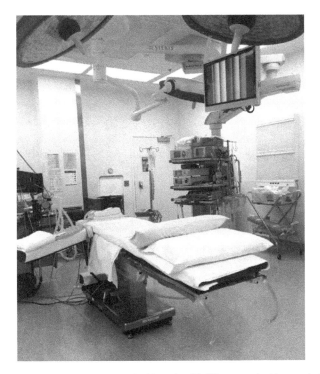

FIGURE 2.5 The intimidating site upon arrival into the OR. (Photo used with permission from Deanna Attai, MD., FACS, David Geffen School of Medicine at UCLA.)

and wearing sterile gloves and gown) and the anesthesiologist (focusing on the head and airway of the patient), anyone else in the room can and should help. The patient bed will be brought up to the edge of the OR bed. Keep in mind there is more to moving individuals safely than pushing/pulling limbs. Take a moment to look down and make sure that both the stretcher or bed the patient is on, and the bed they are being moved to, are locked (Figure 2.6). Whatever problem the patient came into the OR for, it will be exacerbated if they slip down between the two beds and end up on the floor.

Make sure that any tubes, lines, or wires attached to the patient are not wound around the side of a bedrail or wedged between the beds (Figure 2.7). It pays to double-check these things, regardless of your role. Speak up if you notice that something isn't secured or is caught on something.

When everyone is confident that beds are locked and all tubes and lines are accounted for, we turn to anesthesia. Because the anesthesiologist is at the head of the bed managing the airway and able to see the whole picture, they decide when it is time to move the patient and will guide the process, but anyone should speak up if they see a problem.

Some patients are perfectly capable of transferring themselves to the OR table. Even if they can scoot themselves from one bed to the next, keep in mind that

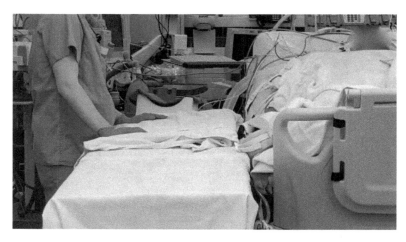

FIGURE 2.6 Beds are brought together to prepare for the move. (Photo used with permission from Ruth Braga, University of Utah.)

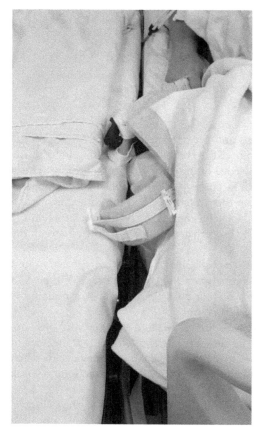

FIGURE 2.7 Watch for anything that may get caught in between the beds. (Photo used with permission from Ruth Braga, University of Utah.)

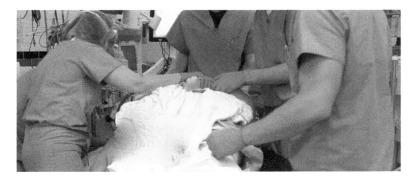

FIGURE 2.8 Everyone assists with positioning when possible. (Photo used with permission from Ruth Braga, University of Utah.)

medications have been given and that OR beds tend to be narrow. Have someone stand next to the OR bed as the patient moves over to provide a stopping point in case the patient scoots too far or doesn't come across as much as they need to in order to be completely on the OR bed (Figure 2.8).

When the patient is safely on the OR bed, a safety strap will be secured over their waist, and arm boards will be attached to the bed (Figure 2.9). This is where nerves can kick in and the patient may need some extra reassurance. Offer this with kind words, an explanation of what is going to happen next, and place a comforting hand on the shoulder, or grab another warm blanket for the patient, especially since the OR is notoriously cold.

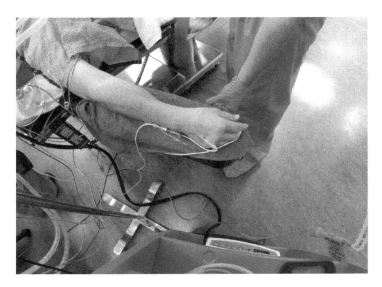

FIGURE 2.9 Armboards should be placed in a natural position for the patient. (Photo used with permission from Ruth Braga, University of Utah.)

Take a moment to consider your patient's position: with masked strangers looming over them, they have been stripped of all personal belongings and written on; they are now barely clothed, nervous, cold, strapped to a narrow table, and medicated. You can't get much more vulnerable than that.

■ TIME-OUT

With the utterance of these words, silence should fall over the team, everyone should stop what they are doing, and one person (usually the circulating nurse) takes the spotlight to perform the time-out. Before anyone touches the patient, we have to double check that we have a few things straight:

1. This really is the patient who we think it is
2. We are all planning on doing the operation that is on this consent (and nothing else)
3. We all agree that left is left, and right is right (if we are supposed to remove, fix, open, etc. the *left* _____, we definitely should not be removing, fixing, opening, etc. the *right* _____) AND that the patient is correctly marked
4. Everyone is aware of the patient's allergies
5. We have everything we need in the room for this operation
6. Antibiotics or other necessary perioperative medications have been given

Although a time-out can vary slightly by institution, it should be standardized. Patients appreciate hearing these things out loud so they know that you know what you are doing. Wrong-site surgery still occurs far too often.

■ HERE WE GO...

Once the patient is situated on the OR table and the time out is complete, anesthesia has the spotlight, taking over key functions for the patient when they go to sleep. If the operation involves general anesthesia (see Chapter 4) a tube goes into the patient's throat after they are appropriately "asleep." If they are being sedated, oxygen goes on, medication goes into the IV, and the snoring begins. From this moment forward, the anesthesiologist, registered nurse anesthetist, anesthesia assistant, or anesthesia resident will be at the head of the bed, constantly monitoring the patient.

Monitoring (see Chapter 14) can mean more than heart rate and blood pressure. If the operation is going to take several hours, the patient may need a urinary catheter inserted, which the nurse or their designee will place once the patient is asleep. Lines may be placed to monitor things such as arterial pressure. Other monitors may watch nerve activity, muscle movement, and blood flow. The patient will be positioned (see Chapter 14) so that access to the surgical site is as direct as possible, and a surgical prep will be placed onto the skin where the incision will be made. That single spot will become the focus for activity until it is time for the patient to be awakened and moved out of the OR. Depending on the procedure, surgical instruments, sponges, suture needles, blades, and injection needles will be counted *at a minimum* before the surgery begins and during closing at the conclusion of the operation.

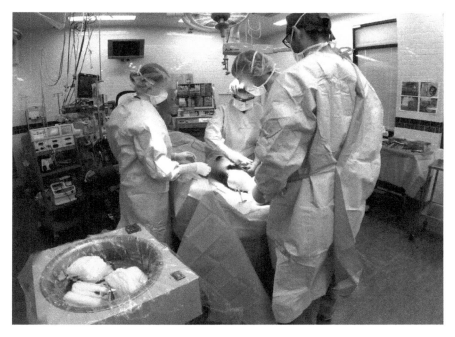

FIGURE 2.10 With the time-out complete, it is time to operate. (Photo used with permission from Ruth Braga, University of Utah.)

■ SCALPEL!

Once the patient is prepped, the surgeon and residents will go out of the operating room to the scrub sink (see Chapter 14). After scrubbing, with fingers pointing to the sky, they will carefully walk into the OR to be gowned and gloved. Sterile cloths, or drapes, will be laid around the operative site on the patient to create a barrier from as many microorganisms as possible. Equipment is plugged in, everything is fired up, and that famous word is uttered: "Scalpel" (Figure 2.10).

■ AND SO IT BEGINS

With a slice of the skin, this finely tuned team works together to accomplish the goal they set out to do: help their patient. As you will learn, each individual has a part to play. Depending on the team (see Chapter 5) in the OR, we may talk, laugh (see Chapter 6), or listen to music (see Chapter 8). Some cases are so fast that the patient is in and out of the room before a nurse has a chance to chart anything. Other cases are so long that they begin one day and finish the next, with replacement teams coming and going.

When the operation is complete, dressings are placed, and every instrument, sponge, blade, and needle is accounted for, anesthesia will reverse the process and wake the patient up. The surgeon will speak to the family or friends who came with the patient, and the nurse will help anesthesia get the patient over to the

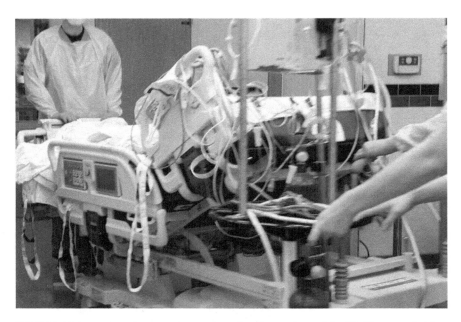

FIGURE 2.11 It can also take a team to move a patient into and out of the OR. (Photo used with permission from Ruth Braga, University of Utah.)

postoperative care unit where they will be monitored closely (Figure 2.11). As soon as the patient is out of the room, it is time to clean up, and if another case is scheduled, set up for the next patient.

■ SPECIAL OCCASIONS: TRAUMA

If you enjoy a good adrenaline rush, then trauma might be the place for you (Figure 2.12). These are the patients who come quickly to the operating room following the briefest of assessments, if any, in the emergency department. There is little regard for clothing in the trauma bay as the trauma shears quickly but safely tear through anything standing between skin and the surgeon. Wedding rings are cut off with special cutters. Jewelry is hastily removed. A nurse or other available staff member gathers the patient's belongings and places them in a bag. This bag will be handed off to the social worker or security, who will have the task of placing the belongings in the hands of an emotional family member or friend.

In trauma, we start at "We Need To Operate" and move to "Here We Go," followed by "Scalpel." The patient usually arrives in the operating room already intubated with multiple bags of blood and IV fluids flowing freely into them, and we generally know very little if anything about this person we are operating on.

Multiple things happen quickly in trauma. I have rushed through the placement of a Foley catheter while a patient was having clothing cut off. I have been soaked with bottles of Betadine prep that were dumped onto a patient by a frantic

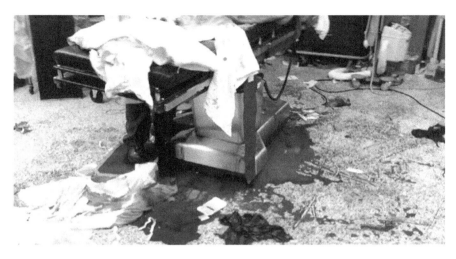

FIGURE 2.12 Trauma can be very exciting—and messy. (Photo used with permission from Ruth Braga, University of Utah.)

resident being told by the attending surgeon to "just get in there." We do our best to count, keep track of items, and maintain sterility. Even in life-or-death situations, we need to keep the patient safe.

Sometimes we manage to get the patient out alive, and sometimes we don't. In the latter case, time of death is called, and the attending surgeon or resident is left with the unfathomable task of walking out of the OR and delivering terrible news. Nurses and other staff do their best to clean up the body. We want to provide an opportunity for the family to see the patient one last time before the body is sent to the morgue. Rules and circumstances will vary, but we try to give the family as much time as they need to say goodbye. If an autopsy is required, the patient is cleaned up, but everything (tubes, lines, IVs, etc.) is carefully left in place.

Any time there is an impending or actual death, it is a requirement in the United States to contact the local organ procurement organization, regardless of circumstance. The patient's medical information is shared and it is determined from there if they are eligible to donate any organ(s). If so, the organ procurement organization takes over the coordination of this process. The knowledge that someone else may benefit from a tragedy may help to ease the pain of loss for family members and friends (Figure 2.13).

Most healthcare providers who encounter death find that there is little time to process what they have just witnessed after a trauma or other difficult case. Regardless of timing or circumstance, providers pull themselves together for the sake of the next patient, and keep moving. Some believe it is a sign of weakness to slow down or acknowledge the experience. It may seem very noble and some may marvel at your resilience, but it all piles on after time. Each of us is affected in our own way. Fortunately, good friends and colleagues help us by being there for us and providing a shoulder to lean on every once in a while (Figure 2.14).

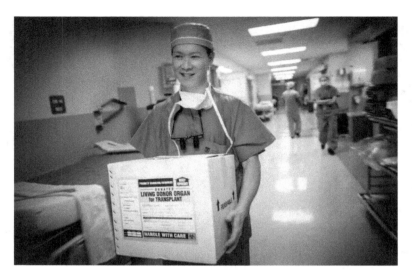

FIGURE 2.13 Transplant brings mixed emotions. To see how the loss of one person's life brings life and joy to another is a humbling experience. (Photo used with permission from Charlie Ehlert, University of Utah.)

■ AND SO IT GOES

The operating room is a fast-paced, fascinating place. Each day brings new situations, and it is not uncommon to hear staff with years of experience say "I have never seen that before!" Whether you end up on the love or hate side of that relationship, it is surely an experience you will never forget.

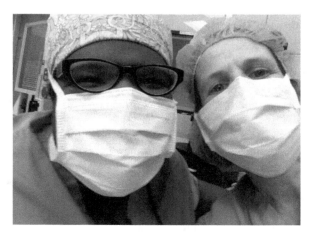

FIGURE 2.14 Dr. Giavonni Lewis and Dr. Amalia Cochran. (Photo used with permission from Amalia Cochran, University of Utah.)

The Myth of the Kind Surgeon

• *Thomas K. Varghese Jr., MD, MS, FACS*

Mythology is the term given to a collection of teachings that belong to a particular group, used to explain the nature of their world and the origins and significance of their ritual practices. The operating room is naturally full of sacred rites dealing with the human condition (good and evil), and human origins (life and death). In this world emerged the flawed hero—the surgeon. How did the classic character traits of the surgeon—the "God complex"—emerge? And is there any place for a kind surgeon?

◼ IN THE BEGINNING

Surgery entails the physical manipulation of a bodily structure to diagnose, prevent, or cure an illness. The sixteenth century French surgeon Ambroise Paré stated that surgery "eliminates that which is superfluous, restores that which has been dislocated, separates that which has been united, joins that which has been divided, and repairs defects of nature."[1]

From the beginning, all surgeons have had to deal with three issues—bleeding, pain, and infection. Early attempts at suturing cuts, amputating mangled limbs, and draining and cauterizing open wounds were for the most part futile as one of the three issues reared its ugly head. Surgery was painful and surgeons were encouraged to be as quick as possible to minimize patient suffering. Brute, efficient force was the norm. There wasn't time for anything else. Surgeries were mainly amputations and removal of external growths. An amazing patient-centered account came in 1811 from the novelist Fanny Burney, who, after being diagnosed with breast cancer, underwent a mastectomy:

> When the dreadful steel was plunged into the breast—cutting through veins—arteries—flesh—nerves—I needed no injunctions not to restrain my cries. I began a scream that lasted unintermittingly during the whole time of my incision—and I almost marvel that it rings not in my Ears still! So excruciating was the agony.[2]

One can imagine the temperament a surgeon needed in this era—detached, oblivious to the blood-curdling screams of their patients, and the ability to come back again and again despite poor outcomes.

In the 1840s, ether emerged as the anesthetic of choice and allowed for the first entries into successful intricate operations in the internal regions of the human body. The added time this afforded allowed for attention to bleeding and minimization of pain. However, increased surgery led to the realization that though patients survived their operations, they were undone by the emergence of dangerous postoperative infections. Overcoming this barrier surprisingly came from two sources—the introduction of meticulous hand washing in 1847 by the Hungarian doctor Ignaz Semmelweis, and the concepts of sterilizing surgical instruments and preventing bacteria from entering the wounds at the time of surgery by Joseph Lister in the 1860s. Lister later implemented the use of sterile gloves to effectively complete his tasks.[3]

With the combination of effective anesthesia and antisepsis, the tide turned. Surgeons began to achieve success in interventions in the body and curing disease. Prestige naturally followed success, and the God-complex began. The public, celebrating successful outcomes where previously there had been none, now embraced surgeons irrespective of their character flaws. The reality, however, was that surgeons were still dealing with life-and-death situations. And in this familiar chaos, historic attitudes prevailed—detachment, confidence bordering on arrogance, and intolerance for the imperfect.

■ THE MODERN ERA

So what turned the tide against the God complex? Surgery in the modern era is a team sport. As survival from surgical interventions has become the norm, attention turned toward other aspects of care. Many of the previously celebrated traits of surgeons are now viewed as outdated and even dangerous. Emotional outbursts, insults, and throwing instruments are no longer tolerated and are considered detrimental to care. Studies emerged demonstrating that good patient-surgeon relationships had a positive impact on outcomes, and that surgeon empathy rather than emotional intelligence was the key driver.[4] Interpersonal dynamics were identified as critically important to performance in the operating room, with linkage of higher risk for death and complications in patients whose surgical teams exhibited less teamwork behaviors.[5,6,7]

Every member of the team has a role in the successful outcome of a surgical intervention. Leadership is an integral component of teamwork, but debate still exists on what particular leadership styles should be embraced in the operating room. Effective surgical leaders support change, encourage speaking up, and act consciously to diminish the power differential between surgeons and other members of the team.[8] A recent study demonstrated that transactional (task-focused) leaders achieve minimum standards, while transformational (team-oriented) leaders inspire performance beyond expectations.[9] In the exploratory study, teams led by transformational surgeons demonstrated a statistically increased rate of information sharing and voice behaviors, which can potentially improve safety and efficiency in the OR.

■ TAKE-HOME POINTS

Despite preliminary studies, many feel that there is no body of literature that guides surgeons in the cultivation of particular behaviors or leadership styles to succeed in the modern era. However, we do not need to wait for "evidence" to learn the best behaviors for a successful career in surgery and life. We've known it all along.

One of my favorite books of all time is Robert Fulghum's *All I Really Need to Know I Learned in Kindergarten*.[10] A truly transformative book, Fulghum emphasized the Kindergartener's Creed in his opening chapter, the secret to leading a remarkable life. The principles of the creed can be adopted by surgeons as follows:

- *Share everything.* Be selfless in praising your team. Share your tips for successful surgical techniques with your students, residents, fellows, and partners.
- *Play fair.* Hold yourself up to the high standards you expect from others. Don't criticize if you don't follow the principles that you preach.
- *Don't hit people.* No-brainer. Plus assault and battery are illegal.
- *Put things back where you found them. Don't take things that aren't yours.* Remember when your mom and kindergarten teacher told you this? They knew what they were talking about.
- *Clean up your own mess. Flush.* Do we need to explain this?
- *Say you're sorry when you hurt somebody.* Especially your patients. We are human. We make mistakes. Take ownership of the same.
- *Wash your hands before you eat.* Wash your hands before you do anything. You don't need to repeat the experiments of the 1860s to know that. Surgeons should have the cleanest hands in the hospital.
- *Warm cookies and cold milk are good for you. Live a balanced life—learn some and think some; and draw and paint and sing and dance and play and work every day some. Take a nap every afternoon.* These are the "take care of yourself" pearls of wisdom. If you are not at your physical and emotional best, you are setting yourself up for failure. Exercise daily. Try yoga. Incorporate relaxation techniques. Though we can't take naps during our workday, it goes without saying that rest and effective sleep can enhance your performance.
- *When you go out into the world, watch out for traffic, hold hands, and stick together.* Develop your team. Your success is highly dependent on it.
- *Wonder. Remember the little seed in the Styrofoam cup: the roots go down and the plant goes up and nobody really knows how or why, but we are all like that.* Successful outcomes in surgery is a recent phenomenon. Embrace the opportunity to work in the modern era, where amazing things can be done on behalf of your patients. There is no debate. We are truly privileged to be surgeons.
- *Goldfish and hamsters and white mice and even the little seed in the Styrofoam cup—they all die. So do we.* Sometimes, despite our best efforts, our patients die. Be honest with family members. Learn from bad outcomes. Improve yourself so that you can help the next patient.

- *Remember the Dick and Jane books, and the first words you learned—the biggest word of all—LOOK.* Learn from every experience, good and bad. Critically analyze your outcomes. Seek opportunities to be kind to everyone.

Being nice is not a sign of weakness. In fact, the kind surgeon is not a myth—success in today's world for your patients, career, and interpersonal development is highly dependent upon it. We close with two quotes that highlight the importance of kindness for surgeons:

> Three things in human life are important. The first is to be kind. The second is to be kind. And the third is to be kind.
> *Henry James*

> Kindness is more important than wisdom, and the recognition of this is the beginning of wisdom.
> *Theodore Isaac Rubin*

■ REFERENCES

1. Porter R. The Greatest Benefit to Mankind: A Medical History of Humanity. New York: WW Norton and Company; 1999. p. 188.
2. Kaplan M. Breast Cancer in 1811: Fanny Burney's Account of Her Mastectomy. The New Jacksonian Blog. Dec 2, 2010. http://newjacksonianblog.blogspot.com/2010/12/breast-cancer-in-1811-fanny-burneys.html (accessed January 11, 2016).
3. Rosen C. Alec Baldwin's 'I Am God' Speech from 'Malice' Is 20 Years Old. The Huffington Post 10/1/2013. http://www.huffingtonpost.com/2013/10/01/alec-baldwin-i-am-god-malice_n_4019992.html (accessed January 11, 2016).
4. Weng HC, Steed JF, Yu SW, et al. The effect of surgeon empathy and emotional intelligence on patient satisfaction. *Adv Health Sci Educ Theory Pract* 2011; 16(5):591–600.
5. Mazzocco K, Peitti DB, Fong KT, et al. Surgical team behaviors and patient outcomes. *Am J Surg* 2009; 197: 678–685.
6. Catchpole K, Mishra A, Handa A, McCulloch P. Teamwork and error in the operating room: analysis of skills and roles. *Ann Surg* 2008; 247(4):699–706.
7. Davenport DL, Henderson WG, Mosca CL, et al. Risk-adjusted morbidity in teaching hospitals correlates with reported levels of communication and collaboration on surgical teams but not with scale measures of teamwork climate, safety climate, or working conditions. *J Am Coll Surg* 2007; 205 (6):778–784.
8. Edmundson AC. Speaking up in the operating room: how team leaders promote learning in interdisciplinary action teams. *J Manage Studies* 2003; 40:1419–1452.
9. Hu Y, Henrickson Parker S, Lipsitz SR, et al. Surgeons' leadership styles and team behavior in the operating room. *J Am Coll Surg* 2016; 222(1):41–51.
10. Fulghum R. *All I Really Need to Know I Learned in Kindergarten.* Ballantine Books; revised edition, May 4, 2004.

Who Are These People?

The Anesthesiologist

- *Christopher J. Behrens, MD*

Historically, the role of the anesthesiologist was limited to the physician who administers anesthesia to suppress pain and consciousness in a patient undergoing surgery. Today, The American Society of Anesthesiologists defines an anesthesiologist as a perioperative physician, the "all-around" physician responsible for providing medical care through all junctures of a patient's surgical course. In the current health care system, in addition to providing pain control and life support functions during and after surgery, anesthesiologists play important roles in preoperative surgical planning and preparation as well as many other aspects of patient care.

■ EDUCATION

At many teaching institutions around the country you may encounter anesthesia residents in training. Anesthesiology residency is a four-year program after medical school requiring one year of internship and three years of anesthesia-specific training. Quick tip for medical students: if you do not enjoy physiology and pharmacology, anesthesiology may not be the right specialty for you. A resident performs the roles and responsibilities of an anesthesiologist under supervision of a staff (fully trained) anesthesiologist. During the operation many of the OR staff may come and go but an anesthesiologist will be present during induction, emergence, and all critical portions of the operation. Anesthesia residents often spend rotations in specialized areas of anesthesia as part of their training including cardiac, transplant, pediatric, regional, ambulatory, and neuroanesthesia, as well as critical care, acute pain, and chronic pain. Following residency, some anesthesiologists will pursue fellowship training in these specialties.

■ THE ANESTHESIOLOGIST'S JOB

The anesthesiologist's job starts prior to surgery with assessment of the patient's medical and surgical history. This may start weeks before a planned operation to allow time for appropriate testing and medical treatment if a patient has complex medical problems. The aim of this preoperative evaluation is to discover risk factors that must be assessed and managed, including acute and chronic diseases of the heart, lungs, kidneys, and liver, allergies, medications, and difficult access to the circulation or airway. Failure to carefully evaluate and manage the patient preoperatively may result in delay of the operation or increased complications during or after the surgery. The preoperative evaluation and plan may be performed by another anesthesia provider weeks before but will be reviewed by the anesthesiologist on the day of the operation. Intraoperatively the objectives of the anesthesiologist for the patient include loss of awareness, pain control, vital sign monitoring and intervention, airway management and breathing, and appropriate hydration with intravascular fluid administration. The anesthesiologist assumes control of the patient's general physiology throughout their operative case.

■ TYPES OF ANESTHESIA

General Anesthesia

If a general anesthesia is planned, on arrival into the operating room the patient will first be placed on appropriate monitors for the procedure. For every anesthetic, the patient's oxygenation, breathing, and circulation are continually monitored as well as temperature if changes are anticipated, intended, or suspected. Monitoring is usually accomplished through use of a pulse oximeter, ECG monitor, blood pressure cuff, and temperature probe. In addition to these standard monitors, some procedures might also require more advanced monitoring and interventions such as a depth of anesthesia monitor, intravascular monitors, and real-time imaging of organs such as the heart with the use of ultrasound. These monitors may be placed before or after initiation of anesthesia (Figure 4.1).

Once the appropriate monitoring is in place, the patient is prepared for the start of anesthesia, which is referred to as "induction." The patient will be asked to breathe 100% oxygen via a plastic mask that is sealed around the mouth and nose. This step is to give the patient an oxygen reserve from the time the patient stops breathing after induction to when the anesthesiologist can safely assist their breathing. Once the patient is pre-oxygenated, anesthesia is initiated, most often with a memory loss medication (induction agent), a fast-acting pain reliever, and a muscle relaxant given through a vein. The patient will lose consciousness and stop breathing very quickly, almost always in less than a minute. At this point, the anesthesiologist may help the patient breathe with the mask used for pre-oxygenation or proceed directly to placing a hollow plastic tube, called an endotracheal tube, into the trachea, the structure connecting the patient's mouth to the lungs. To place the endotracheal tube, a laryngoscope is used. A laryngoscope is a blunt metal blade with a bright light on the end, used to push the tongue out of the way and light up the opening of the trachea. When endotracheal tube placement is

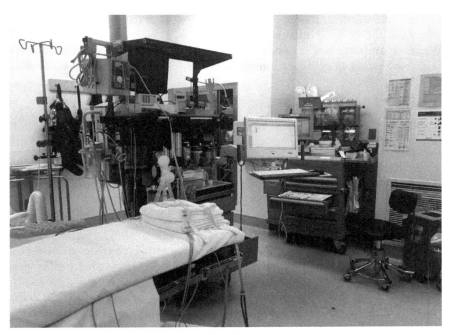

FIGURE 4.1 Monitoring equipment for anesthesia. (Photo used with permission from Deanna Attai, UCLA.)

confirmed, the tube is secured in place and breathing is assisted or taken over for the patient. If the anesthesiologist anticipates a difficult airway, the endotracheal tube might be placed with the patient under light sedation with local anesthetic while the patient remains breathing on their own.

During the operation, the anesthesiologist maintains anesthesia and preserves stable heart and lung function. Most commonly, anesthesia is maintained with a vapor inhaled through the lungs, which travels through the bloodstream and acts on the central nervous system. Maintenance of anesthesia may involve the use of a number of different drugs and fluids, especially when the operation is associated with major interruption of blood flow or major blood loss.

After the operation is complete, if it's possible for the patient to breathe without assistance the anesthesiologist will reverse the effects of muscle relaxants and anesthetics and remove the endotracheal tube. Awakening from anesthesia is referred to as *emergence*. If the patient requires continued breathing support, the anesthesiologist may decide to leave the endotracheal tube in. In either event, depending upon the intensity of postoperative care required, the anesthesiologist transports the patient to either the postoperative care unit or an intensive care unit. During this recovery period, the post-anesthesia care unit or critical care nurses may administer drugs to relieve pain, control blood pressure, and stabilize organ function.

Depending on the type and duration of procedure being performed, the anesthesiologist may choose a technique other than general anesthesia. Other types of anesthetics include monitored anesthesia care, regional anesthesia, neuraxial anesthesia, or a combination of these techniques. Oxygenation, ventilation, and perfusion must still be monitored with alternative anesthetic techniques and there is always a possibility of transitioning to general anesthesia during the procedure.

Monitored Anesthesia Care

Monitored anesthesia care (often referred to as MAC) differs from general anesthesia by allowing the patient to continue breathing under their own power and keeping the patient able to respond to touch or verbal stimuli. This is usually accomplished with IV sedative medications or slow, less aggressive infusions of the same medications used to induce general anesthesia. Vapor inhaled anesthetics are rarely used, as they are pungent and unpleasant to breathe spontaneously.

Regional Anesthesia

Regional anesthesia involves injection of a local anesthetic around major nerves to block pain from a large region of the body. The nerves are found using anatomic landmark, nerve stimulator, or ultrasound-guided techniques. For example, a supraclavicular block to the brachial plexus will provide anesthesia to the majority of the arm. Nerve blocks are most commonly used for procedures on the hands, arms, legs, or face. The choice to perform regional anesthesia depends on the patient's ability to tolerate the block, to tolerate the operating room environment, and the length and location of the procedure. Regional anesthesia can also be performed after an operation to provide postoperative pain relief.

Neuraxial Anesthesia

Neuraxial anesthesia includes injection or continuous infusions of local anesthetics in close proximity to the spinal cord. A spinal anesthetic is often used for lower abdominal, pelvic, rectal, or lower extremity surgery. This type of anesthetic involves injecting a single dose of local anesthetic agent directly into the spinal cord fluid in the lower back, causing numbness in the lower body.

Epidural or Caudal Anesthetic

An epidural or caudal anesthetic is similar to a spinal anesthetic, and is also commonly used for surgery of the lower limbs and during labor and childbirth. This type of anesthesia involves continual infusion of drugs through a thin catheter that has been placed into the space that surrounds the spinal cord in the lower back, causing numbness in the abdomen and lower body. The advantage of an epidural or caudal anesthetic over spinal is that it allows adjustable anesthetic doses for a long duration. However, epidural and caudal anesthetics can be unreliable in their spread and strength of blocking the nerves due to the complexity of the spaces into which the infusions are entering.

The anesthesiologist is a great resource for learning about airway management, pharmacology, and complex physiology while patients are in the operating room. Their role is central to the safety of the surgical patient before, during, and after their operation.

The Nurse Anesthetist

* *Clive Thirkill, MSN, CRNA*

I remember getting a call at 2:00 in the morning from the obstetrician saying that we had to rush to the OR with an emergency postpartum hemorrhage. Just hours before that, I placed a labor epidural in this same patient to help relieve her pain during labor, in anticipation for her first child. I remember the proud look on the new father's face as they transferred the family to the postpartum unit. Upon hearing the news that we must rush to surgery, I saw the same father anxiously waiting outside the OR, his face much different this time! I assured him that his wife was in good hands. The OR staff were all busily preparing for emergency surgery. I noticed the patient was afraid and in a state of shock. I grabbed her hand and explained that I would have to place her under general anesthesia so the surgeons could control the bleeding, and I would be by her side and help her get through this unexpected event. I continued to reassure her until she was comfortably asleep under anesthesia. This story exemplifies how I unite my experience as a bedside nurse with my expertise in anesthesia—a unique skill set possessed by Certified Registered Nurse Anesthetists (CRNAs).

CRNAs are highly trained providers of anesthesia. We are first and foremost nurses. Our training begins with a bachelor's degree in nursing, and all CRNAs must have critical care experience prior to their anesthesia training. This bedside care experience helps CRNAs to connect with their patients on a personal level. It has been invaluable to me as I try to ease the (appropriate) anxiety most patients experience before going to surgery. In addition to our critical care experience, all CRNA programs are between 28 and 36 months, leading to a masters or doctoral degree. Following completion of degree requirements, a rigorous board examination must be passed to ensure competence, and for the safety of the public. These are the entry-level requirements to begin the practice of anesthesia as a nurse.

Anesthesia was first practiced by nurses on the battlefields of the Civil War in 1860 and became the first nursing specialty in the United States. Currently, 38 million anesthetics are provided by CRNAs in the United States each year. At many hospitals where CRNAs practice in a team with anesthesiologists (Figure 4.2). This partnership adds a unique quality to the patients we serve, while keeping safety our top priority.

Anesthesia is 50 times safer today than it was in the 1980s. Practicing anesthesia in teams has the added benefit of making anesthesia even safer for our patients. CRNAs communicate closely with our anesthesiologist colleagues, freeing them to identify risks, mitigate those risks, and provide for a smooth recovery from anesthesia in the recovery room. You will always see an anesthesiologist present during the key moments of anesthesia, including induction, emergence, and placement of invasive lines.

In my anesthesia training I was taught to plan for a smooth anesthetic but always be prepared for the worst. In the example of the postpartum hemorrhage, I had previously prepared myself for any emergency. As the OR staff were busy with the tasks of preparing for surgery, I was free to attend to the patient's fears. My

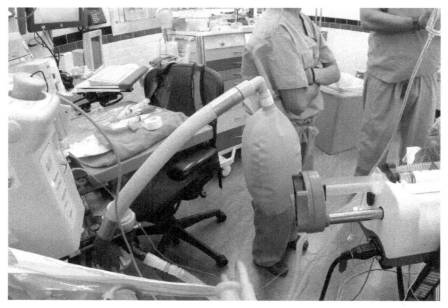

FIGURE 4.2 CRNA working alongside the anesthesiologist. (Photo used with permission from Ruth Braga, University of Utah.)

years of bedside nursing experience made me remember that my duty was not only to administer anesthesia, but also to care holistically for patients and their families.

From Medical Student to Surgeon

• *Brian J. Gavitt, MD, MPH*

A surgical team at an academic medical center is composed of individuals at multiple levels in their training and careers. There is a specific surgical hierarchy in the operating room and it is important for everyone to understand this, especially during cases involving critically ill patients (Figure 4.3).

■ EDUCATION

The clinical training to become a general surgeon is five years long, following medical school. Other surgical specialties such as obstetrics and gynecology, neurosurgery, or otolaryngology have training that ranges from four to six years. Choosing what type of physician to become is a lengthy process that usually starts during undergraduate training, where premedical students will follow (or "shadow") senior physicians to better understand what different specialists do. Premedical

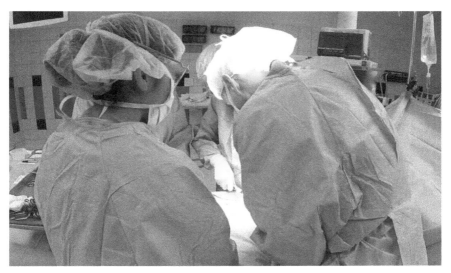

FIGURE 4.3 The attending operates and teaches multiple individuals simultaneously. (Photo used with permission from Ruth Braga, University of Utah.)

students have no formal training in OR etiquette or procedure and will usually need specific instructions from the OR nursing and scrub staff on where to stand and how to avoid contaminating the sterile field. If you are a premedical student, I can't emphasize enough to you—*please* ask questions when you are observing in the OR so that you don't breach etiquette or have a negative impact on the safety of the patient.

In medical school, students typically begin to scrub for cases during their third year. Medical students receive varying amounts of training on how to properly scrub and maintain sterility, so assuming they know proper sterile technique can be dangerous. Medical students rotate through various specialties during their clinical years, so they will have limited time and experience in the operating room. They will usually help the surgical team with retraction during cases and generally focus on learning the operative indications and anatomy. Medical students are commonly tasked with closing the incision at the end of the case. Expect medical students to struggle initially with wound closure, and keep in mind how you appreciated the patience of your senior colleagues early in your training.

When a medical student graduates, they are officially referred to as "doctor," and enter a residency training program. Residency is when physicians become specialists in different areas of medicine such as a family practice, pediatrics, surgery, or radiology. The clinical training to become a surgeon, as noted above, generally lasts five years. First-year residents, referred to as *interns*, typically spend most of their time outside the OR learning how to manage patients before and after surgery. When interns do come to the operating room they are closely supervised by more-senior doctors and are focused on learning basic surgical techniques. The nursing and scrub staff in the OR can play a tremendous role in shaping these future surgeons by helping them learn the names of instruments and also the safe handling and passing of instruments. It is critically important for residents to learn early how to guard needles and safely pass sharps so that it becomes habit even (and especially) during stressful OR cases.

After completing their internship, residents in their second and third years of residency are referred to as *junior residents*. Junior residents will scrub most of the bread-and-butter cases for their specialty and help supervise medical students and interns. Residents in their fourth year of training are typically referred to as *senior residents*, and residents in their final year of surgical training are called *chief residents*. Senior and chief residents will typically scrub for the more complex cases in the operating room and are also tasked with overseeing the rest of the resident team. Senior and chief residents are sometimes entrusted to take a junior resident through a case as a teacher, but today, with the emphasis on patient safety, the attending is expected to be present. It is not uncommon for senior and chief residents to have to field multiple pages and phone calls while scrubbed in for surgery. It is helpful to remember that residents are functionally expected to be in multiple places at once—operating, managing floor and ICU patients, as well as seeing and staffing consults. It can be frustrating to the OR staff to help with returning pages, but this generally speeds cases along and allows the team to function more efficiently.

After completing a surgical residency many surgeons choose to subspecialize into a more focused practice. These subspecialty programs are called *fellowships*. Fellows are focused on learning the complex nuances of their subspecialty and generally practice relatively independently under the direction of a mentoring attending surgeon. Fellows will often complete cases as the attending of record and are responsible for teaching and directly supervising residents in the operating room.

Finally, the most senior member of a surgical team is the *surgical attending* or *consultant*. The surgical attending is the individual ultimately responsible for the care of the patient in the operating room and makes the final decisions on all care provided to the patient. Depending on the type of case in the OR, there may be multiple attending surgeons present for a given operation, and ideally the interaction is collegial and allows for a safe and efficient operation for the patient. Cases with multiple attending surgeons present a particular challenge for OR staff in terms of setup and expectations, so extra preparation, extra communication, and extra patience is fundamental during these events.

Surgical training is lengthy and rigorous because of the amount of medical knowledge and technical skill that surgeons must have to care for patients. Surgeons have to be able to operate under both ideal and difficult conditions, and they also must know when offering an operation is unlikely to help a patient (and therefore not offer that operation).

Surgery is both an incredibly challenging and an incredibly rewarding career because of the complexity of what surgeons do, and because we are entrusted by patients and families to "fix" something about their health. Most importantly, surgeons cannot function alone; effective teamwork with the rest of the surgical team is mandatory for successful outcomes for our patients.

The Role of the Resident in the Operating Room

• *Lara Senekjian, MD, MAT*

In the OR, the main goal of the resident is to learn how to perform the operation while providing the best possible care for the patient. The resident is always under the supervision of the attending surgeon, but as the resident's skill and knowledge improves he or she is given more independence. Before we take the patient into the OR, the resident will ensure that the correct surgery is going to be performed on the correct patient. Under the direction or with the assistance of the attending surgeon, residents identify if and when a patient needs surgery. It is important to discuss the risks, benefits, and alternatives of the surgery with the patient. This is referred to as the *informed consent process*. Prior to the OR, the resident also ensures that all required paperwork is completed and any necessary labs or imaging are done. Often this requires writing or updating a history and physical.

Prior to the patient arriving to the OR, the resident will review relevant labs and imaging. One of the resident's jobs is to have the x-rays or scans pulled up on a computer monitor in the OR. If the surgical plan is unclear to the resident, they will ask the attending for clarification as a learning exercise and to optimize the patient's care and safety. A resident will often speak with the attending to learn how to do the operation as well as how to troubleshoot if there is an event in the operating room. It is important that the resident comes to the operating room completely prepared, with an understanding of the attending's surgical plan. As the resident becomes more advanced, the attending may challenge them to create their own surgical plan, and will review it with them prior to surgery. The resident also is responsible for verifying that all supplies that may be needed in the surgery are available.

Once the patient arrives in the OR, the resident helps the nurse place the patient on the operating room table. A time-out is conducted to verify the patient's planned surgery, the indications for it, any drug allergies that the patient has, and the antibiotic plan. The time-out must include the attending surgeon, the anesthesiologist, and the circulating nurse. Once the anesthesiologist puts the patient to sleep, the resident will help get the patient positioned correctly, place the Foley catheter if one is needed, and gather appropriate supplies. If the case is laparoscopic, the resident will help to get the screens into an appropriate position, or may tuck the arms if this helps to position the patient appropriately. Once the patient is safely positioned, the resident will prepare the surgical site, though some attending surgeons prefer to do this, and sometimes circulating nurses may offer to help.

After the surgical scrub, the operative team gowns, gloves, and then drapes the patient (Figure 4.4). The way the patient is draped depends on the surgery to be performed and may be strongly influenced by attending preference. The resident should be familiar with the surgical plan to ensure appropriate draping.

After all of these preparatory steps, the operation can finally start; as a new observer in the OR you may sometimes wonder if the team spends more time

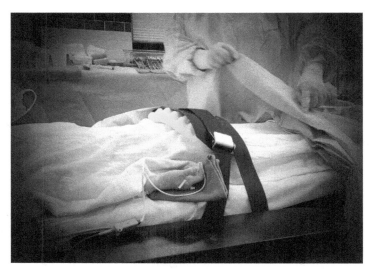

FIGURE 4.4 Resident carefully draping the patient. (Photo used with permission from Ruth Braga, University of Utah.)

preparing for the case than performing the actual surgery. The resident will either assist the attending or the attending will assist the resident, depending on resident skill and seniority. If the resident is very capable, they may be assisted by a second resident to complete the surgery or may be given responsibility for teaching a junior resident how to perform an operation (Figure 4.5). Throughout the surgery, the resident should ask questions to ensure that they are progressing appropriately through the steps of the operation and that they are effectively using their technical skills. Residents expect the attending to teach during the surgery, and a resident will simultaneously also teach the medical student or junior resident about the anatomy and physiology of the patient, as well as about the surgery being performed (Figure 4.6).

When the operation is complete, the resident will close the patient's skin and place dressings as appropriate. The resident helps to move the patient back onto their bed and ensure they are taken from the operating room in a safe manner. The resident often has the responsibility for completion of the brief operative note and dictation of the operative report. The resident also write orders for the patient's care. Finally, the resident makes sure the patient is following an expected postoperative course by checking on the patient after surgery as appropriate to ensure that an urgent or emergent return to the OR is not necessary and that the patient's postoperative course is as expected.

The resident has a unique dual role in the operating room. While the resident is a doctor who has graduated from medical school, they are also still a learner who is in training. The broad responsibilities of the resident highlight these two sets of responsibilities—the resident is accountable for the safety of the patient as a physician, and also needs to learn to be a safe surgeon.

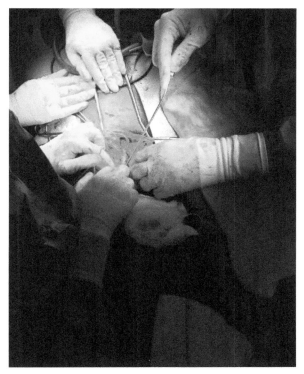

FIGURE 4.5 Many hands at work. (Photo used with permission from Sarah Bryczkowski, Rutgers New Jersey Medical School.)

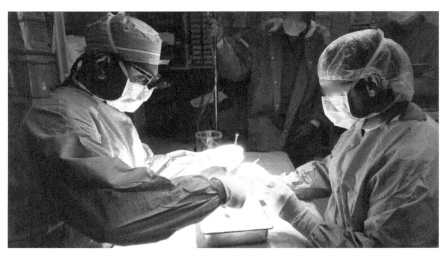

FIGURE 4.6 Transplant teaching. (Photo used with permission from University of Utah Health Sciences Center Transplant Team.)

How to Be a Superstar Medical Student in the Operating Room

• *Madeline B. Torres, MD*

Medical students are an essential part of the surgery team; they serve as the eyes and ears of the team. They are also excellent patient advocates in and out of the operating room. As a medical student, the demands on your time are very different from the demands on residents and faculty, and this fosters a very different patient relationship. Medical students vary by their level of experience and how far along they are in their training. Most commonly, third and fourth year medical students are found in the wards and the OR, as opposed to the first and second year medical students who are cooped up in the classroom.

Depending on your comfort level and prior experience in the OR, your role may vary from helping to set up and retract to first-assisting a case if no other qualified first assistant is available. However, the first and most important role of the medical student is to learn. Learning goes beyond the anatomy, physiology, and technical skills one can learn in the OR. Learning starts with meeting the patient in the pre-op holding area, introducing yourself, then helping to take the patient back to the OR. The OR can be an intimidating place for patients—just like it is for medical students—and having a familiar face present helps ease anxiety. The following is by no means a complete list of the things medical students can help with in the operating room, but is meant to serve as a general guide for medical students and everyone who works with them in the OR. They are things you can help with at the different stages.

■ BEFORE THE PATIENT ENTERS THE OPERATING ROOM

1. Make sure you write your name on the board upon entering the OR.
2. Introduce yourself to the nurse circulator and the surgical technician; ask if you should get your gloves for the case and make sure they have enough gowns for you to have one too.
3. Pull up any pertinent imaging on the computer screen for the attending surgeon and residents to review before and during the surgery.

■ ONCE THE PATIENT IS IN THE OPERATING ROOM, BUT STILL LYING ON THE STRETCHER

1. Hold the door open to help get the patient stretcher into the OR.
2. If you feel comfortable with it, help transfer the patient to the OR table. If you are not comfortable, you can always help hold the feet while you learn how to help move patients (Figure 4.7).
3. During the transfer, if you notice that something is caught or the bed is not locked, speak up. Patient safety comes first, and the patient and team will thank you.
4. If you aren't sure how you can help, just ask.

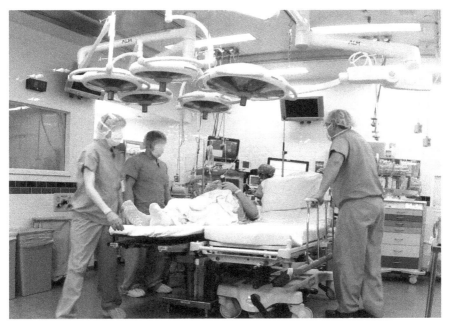

FIGURE 4.7 Two medical students prepare to assist the patient to move over to the OR table. (Photo used with permission from Ruth Braga, University of Utah.)

■ ONCE THE PATIENT IS ON THE OR TABLE

1. Make sure there is someone standing at the bedside to ensure safety of the patient. We can't have patients falling off of the OR bed.
2. Take the stretcher out of the OR and "park" it in a nearby spot.
3. Help place the SCDs (sequential compression devices) on the patient's legs after you explain to him/her what you are doing. Be sure to plug the devices in and turn them on.
4. Help keep the patient covered with warm blankets.
5. Help position the patient; ask the circulating nurse and/or resident what you can help with because you don't want to be "that" medical student who makes assumptions about positioning the patient.
6. If hair needs to be shaved from your patient, ask for the clippers and shave at the site where incision will be. If you've never shaved a patient before, ask for guidance.
7. If someone else is shaving the patient, put gloves on and get tape to collect the remaining hair.
8. Will the patient need a urinary catheter placed? If you have been trained, ask to place it.
9. If you are comfortable and the team and your facility approve it, you may prep the patient.
10. Participate in the time-out. If something is said that doesn't seem right, speak up. Patient safety is first, and this is one place you can be the MVP.

11. If you find yourself with nothing to do while the patient is being placed to sleep, hold their hand and help to make them comfortable. They'll really appreciate your kindness.

■ WHEN THE PATIENT IS PREPPED AND DRAPED

Scrub in. If you haven't done this before, get someone knowledgeable to coach you through the process (Figure 4.8).

■ YOU'RE SCRUBBED IN, NOW WHAT?

1. Don't break the sterile field.
2. Pay attention. Be mindful and engaged. Ask questions during the noncritical portions of the case.
3. You may be asked to retract, cut sutures, tie knots, and maybe even to help close the incision.
4. Once you are more comfortable, you'll be able to assist more easily. When you are new to the OR it can be really hard to anticipate what steps are next. The more time you spend scrubbed in, the easier this becomes.

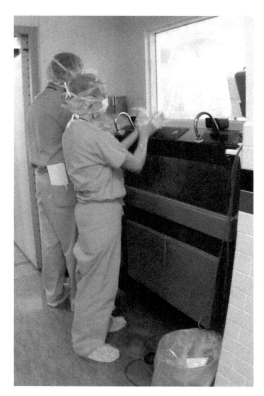

FIGURE 4.8 Medical students scrubbing in (but forgot to put goggles down-just ask the nurse to assist you if this happens). (Photo used with permission from Ruth Braga, University of Utah.)

■ SURGERY IS OVER, NOW WHAT?

1. Grab warm blankets and a clean gown and help cover the patient and keep them warm.
2. Help take extra leads, the bovie pad, and other attachments off the patient. If you aren't sure, ask the circulator or anesthesia. If you remove the bovie grounding pad, make sure to announce that the site looks okay (or if it doesn't, announce that too, so the team knows and can document appropriately).
3. Help transfer the patient back to the stretcher or to their inpatient bed.
4. Write the brief operative note; ask the anesthesia resident/attending how much fluid the patient received, the estimated blood loss, if any urine was measured. All of these things help make your resident's life easier.
5. Accompany the patient to PACU or to the ICU and make sure they are safe.
6. Do post-op checks at approximately two hours and eight hours after the surgery is over. Is the patient's pain controlled? Are they making urine? Are they having terrible nausea and vomiting? Are their vitals okay? Reporting back on these things to your resident shows them that you really care about your patient (because you do).

Remember, the role of the medical student goes beyond learning the basic anatomy, physiology, and surgical skills needed. The role of the medical student in the operating room is to be a patient advocate, a team player, and most importantly an open-minded learner willing to learn from every member of the highly trained team that participates in the care of the patient in this very special place called the OR. We are fortunate to be part of this process.

The Operating Room: View from a Physician Assistant

• *Crystal D. Webb, PA-C*

The operating room is one of my favorite places to be. I enjoy the music and the silence, the ability to work with my hands while not touching a keyboard, and the conversation and educational experience that time in the OR allows that day-to-day tasks do not.

I also enjoy the raw sense of humor that seems to be characteristic of most operating rooms. The unfiltered conversation that flows so freely is a breath of fresh air from the rehearsed, stale, professional discussions in other clinical settings. This is a place where you truly get to know your peers and begin to connect on a deeper level that develops your overall relationships (and sometimes gives you leverage).

First, I find it helpful to know which areas are considered pre-op, recovery, and post-op. Some hospitals house this area all together, some separate, and some far apart. If you do not know, ask someone to point you in the right direction. The OR nurse manager, the charge nurse, or the OR front desk staff are typically happy to help, as they do not want you messing anything up. While you're at it, make sure you ask where the locker room is and how to get scrubs.

Upon entering the operating room area, there is usually a red line on the ground and a large sign stating that only OR attire is allowed past this point. Pay attention, but don't be discouraged if you get yelled at because you forgot to put on your hat. It is not the first time this has happened and it likely won't be the last. Most hats, masks, and booties (shoe covers) are at every entry point into the OR area. Prior to entering, make a checklist in your head of what you may need. If it is your responsibility, did you bring, sign, and update the H&P? When was the last time you drank water? When was the last time you emptied your bladder? Will x-rays be taken during surgery? If yes, then you need to have lead. What is lead? Those ridiculously heavy, typically sparkly, armor-like aprons that you will see some of the staff wearing in order to shield themselves from x-rays during certain surgery.

If you plan on scrubbing in, the first thing to do is to meet the scrub tech and the circulating nurse in your assigned operating room. If you are really savvy, you will write your full name and credentials on the white board. Always ask if you can get your own gown and gloves for the case. If you don't know where they are located, ask.

Become familiar with the surgical instruments your surgeon uses. Know what they like—curved versus straight scissors, tapered versus cutting needles. Often there will be different equipment brands, so make sure to familiarize yourself with each so as to not confuse them. If a sales rep is available for a particular product or equipment, do your best to learn everything you can from them in a brief amount of time.

Learn how the surgeon prefers to prep and drape the patient. While you are standing around waiting for anesthesia to intubate the patient, make sure the scrub tech has the appropriate drapes. Many times the circulating nurse will prepare the surgical site, but may appreciate if you offer your assistance (ask before you assume). Once gowned and gloved you should help the surgical tech drape the patient appropriately if needed.

There will likely be several different types of soaps and sanitizing gels available for scrubbing (Figure 4.9). It truly is personal preference, but trust me: anything with iodine is hard on your skin. You always need to scrub (yes, the full five minutes or the brush stroke method) initially. For all subsequent scrubs, you are allowed to use the sanitizing gel unless you have just eaten, gone out for a smoke, or used the restroom, in which case you must scrub again using water.

After you have scrubbed, it is time to gown and glove. Typically the surgical tech will assist you with both, but if he or she is busy you should know how to do it yourself. For me, this was one of the biggest technical obstacles I faced. I have had a scrub tech watch me fail four times (after the surgeon had already started) before I was able to gown and glove myself, so practice when you can.

During the surgery, always try to think two steps ahead of the surgeon you are working with. Constantly have a lap or Raytech (sterile absorbent cloths) (Figure 4.10)

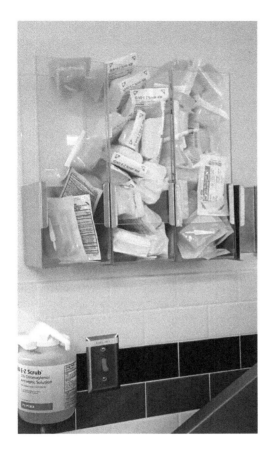

FIGURE 4.9 The variety of soaps/scrub brushes you may see. (Photo used with permission from Ruth Braga, University of Utah.)

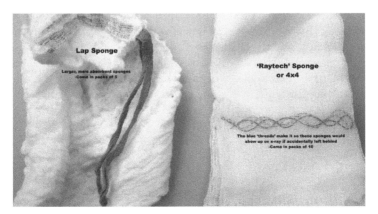

FIGURE 4.10 A close-up sponge comparison. (Photo used with permission from Ruth Braga, University of Utah.)

in hand to wipe or dab if needed. Always make sure suction is available to assist in visualizing the site by suctioning the smoke from burning flesh, or suctioning blood (unless you are in a burn OR—then your effort is usually futile). Continuously check to make sure that there is enough light on the area of focus. Sometimes moving the lights is like a game of Tetris and may cause frustration for you and your surgeon. Sometimes the frustration can result in some salty language, either from them or from.

To become a PA, the application process for school is rigorous and admissions are highly competitive. A minimum of two years of college coursework is required, often including prerequisites in chemistry, physiology, anatomy, microbiology, and anatomy. Many programs also expect prior hands-on patient care experience from applicants; the "average" PA student has a bachelor's degree and three years of healthcare experience before they start PA school. PA school is usually three academic years and results in award of a master's degree. The education process is a combination of classroom instruction and more than 2000 hours of clinical rotations. After graduation, you must pass a certification exam to become eligible for licensing, after which you may indicate that you are a PA-C (Physician Assistant-Certified). Unlike MDs, who are required to do residencies to become certified in a specific field, postgraduate training for PAs is entirely voluntary and has both advantages and disadvantages. These residency programs include special training in surgery, although this is not a requirement to work as surgical PA.

As a PA working in the OR, you will have many different duties. You have a unique job of assuring that most aspects of surgery, including paperwork, are complete, but at the same time you must be able to do specialty procedures such as suturing, cutting, drilling, and harvesting (veins or skin) that a scrub tech cannot. Patience and practice are the key to excelling in these areas. The final duties of a PA during a case include assuring the right dressing is placed correctly and helping anesthesia and nursing transfer the patient back to the gurney. Once the patient is taken to Post-Anesthesia Care Unit, a brief operative report needs to be completed.

There are those to whom the OR does not "speak." There is usually a love or hate relationship. But for those of us who do enjoy extremes of temperature, awkward instrument holding, and the challenge of constant variations in patients (not one single patient has read the anatomy book from cover to cover), it gives you a purpose. You will never experience something so raw and delicate as that patient on the table, trusting you with not just their scars, but their life and future.

The OR Staff

• *Karen Porter, BSN, RN*

The circulating nurse, surgical tech, and health care assistant are the primary, consistent roles that you will see in the operating room setting. Some facilities may have specialty teams such as a heart team, transplant team, etc. as surgeries become more complicated and equipment and instruments become more special-ized, but the core individuals are stable even among these specialized teams.

■ THE CIRCULATOR

The circulator is a registered nurse who is dedicated to caring for one surgical patient at a time. To become a registered nurse, education programs range from 18 months to 4+ years to earn an associate's or bachelor's degree in nursing. There is a national trend for the circulator to be Bachelor's degree prepared.

The circulator has two key roles: to ensure safe delivery of surgical care, and to be a patient advocate. They coordinate patient care with other members of the surgical team from the pre-op area throughout the operative phase and until deliv-ery to the recovery area or the ICU. The circulator ensures that the OR suite is prepared prior to the patient arriving. The appropriate bed, positioning devices, equipment, and medications need to be organized and in place for the surgery. Next, the circulator has a pre-op visit with the patient. They assess the patient and ensure that all paperwork is in order and that any operative questions are addressed. Once the OR suite is ready and the patient is in the room, the circulator often assists with anesthesia induction (Figure 4.11). The circulator also has the responsibility of guiding the "time-out" and making sure that no new information is discovered during the time-out process that changes equipment or care needs for the patient.

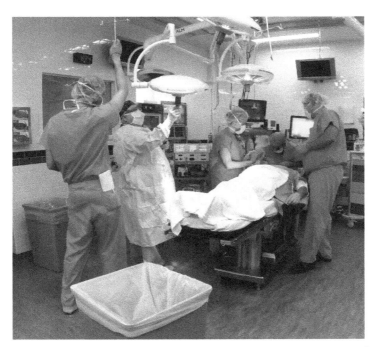

FIGURE 4.11 The nurse remains nearby during intubation. (Photo used with permission from Ruth Braga, University of Utah.)

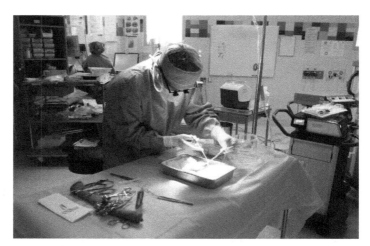

FIGURE 4.12 Once things have settled, the RN documents activity in the OR, maintains the count, and monitors for breaks in sterility. (Photo used with permission from the University of Utah Health Sciences Center Transplant Team.)

Throughout the case, the circulator functions outside of the sterile area in the operating room. Because they are not up at the sterile field and can see the full picture, the circulator assists with monitoring to make sure sterility is never compromised. The circulator also completes all of the OR documentation (this is the very not-glamorous part of the job) (Figure 4.12) and coordinates care of the patient if there is any radiography needed or specimens to be sent. Upon successful completion of surgical counts and wound closure, the circulator will assist anesthesia with extubation and delivery of the patient to the recovery area (Figure 4.13).

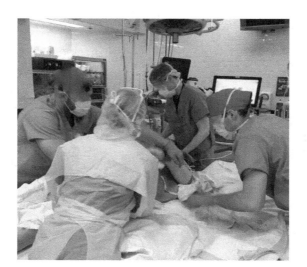

FIGURE 4.13 Nurse moves the patient with the other members of the team. (Photo used with permission from Ruth Braga, University of Utah.)

Because the circulator is outside of the sterile field, they often assume responsibility for relaying telephone messages and answering pages for team members who are scrubbed in. This enables the surgical team members to continue caring for other patients while in the OR without compromising the safety or the needs of the patient currently in the OR. For example, if the OR phone rings during induction, the circulator definitely isn't going to step away to answer it at this critical point. In addition, some surgeons will help the circulator and other team members by declaring certain high-risk portions of procedures as "no outside communication" times. This allows all team members to focus explicitly on the patient in the operating room for that time.

■ THE SCRUB TECHNICIAN

The "scrub," who may be an RN or a surgical technologist, assists the surgeon throughout the surgery. Surgical tech programs vary in duration from nine months to a two-year associate's degree. Scrub techs have specialized knowledge in sterile technique, surgical equipment, and surgical procedures.

The scrub technician is responsible for gathering instruments and supplies used during the case and ensuring that the sterility of the procedure is maintained (Figure 4.14). The scrub should have knowledge of the case that is to be performed and communicate with the surgical team to ensure that all needed supplies and instruments are available. Unlike the circulator, the scrub is in the sterile area and is scrubbed in to the case. The scrub handles all sterile supplies and instruments. They set up the sterile field for the surgical team (Figure 4.15), including medications, and organize all of the surgical instruments. Scrubs may also be assigned to specific teams. Specialized scrubs readily anticipate surgeon needs and are able to teach case specifics to new staff (Figure 4.16). The scrub performs the surgical counts and participates in the time-out to verify that all required equipment is

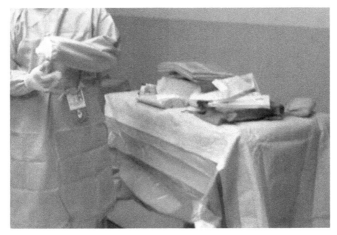

FIGURE 4.14 With all items opened on the back table, the scrub technician scrubs, gowns, and gloves themselves to set up for the surgery. (Photo used with permission from Ruth Braga, University of Utah.)

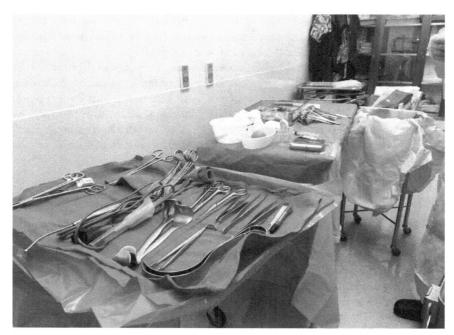

FIGURE 4.15 Completed setup, ready to begin. (Photo used with permission from Deanna Attai, David Geffen School of Medicine at UCLA.)

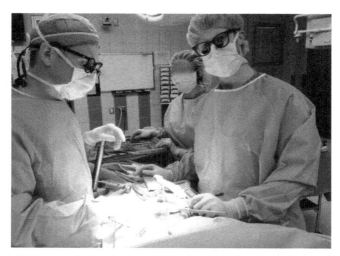

FIGURE 4.16 The scrub technician is always in tune, listening, anticipating, and watching for what is needed next. (Photo used with permission from the University of Utah Health Sciences Center Transplant Team.)

present in the operating room. The scrub will assist with every step from draping the patient to preparing dressings for closure; once the patient leaves the room, they prepare the instruments to be cleaned and processed.

■ THE HEALTHCARE ASSISTANT

The healthcare assistant (HCA) is a vastly different role in the OR than on the floors. The HCA role varies by institution, but these individuals work under the direction of the circulating RN. They may have previous experience as a Certified Nursing Assistant (CNA), and many are enrolled in a nursing or other healthcare education program.

The HCA may be responsible for tasks such as preparing the OR suite for surgery, cleaning the OR, stocking supplies, and gathering the required equipment for each case. They may be responsible for transporting patients, delivering specimens to pathology, and picking up blood products at the blood bank. If they have been trained, an HCA may assist with prepping the patient skin, or scrubbing in and assisting with retraction. Their role is vital to the OR. Because the variety of supplies and items in the operating room is so vast, they are an excellent resource for questions. Their specialized knowledge of equipment and beds is invaluable (Figure 4.17).

Together, the circulator, the scrub technician, and the HCA work closely as the "in the OR" team, communicate what they need, ask questions if they need clarification, and help one another to assist the surgeon and anesthesia with caring for the patient.

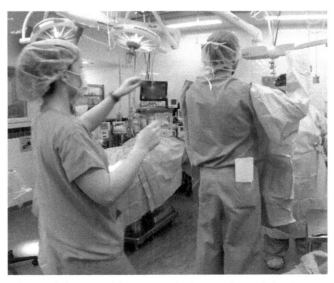

FIGURE 4.17 The HCA helps around the room, gathering supplies, assisting the nurse and team as needed. (Photo used with permission from Ruth Braga, University of Utah.)

The Perfusionist

• *Jennie O'Shea, BS, CCP*

A perfusionist will usually be found in an OR where a cardiac procedure is being performed. The perfusionist is an individual trained to operate equipment that reroutes the flow of human blood from the veins to outside the body, and back into the arteries. A perfusionist spends the majority of their day in the operating room but their responsibilities may take them to the ICU, cardiac catheter lab, emergency room, and even on local and long-range transportation of critically ill patients.

■ EDUCATION

There are currently approximately 3500 perfusionists working in the United States. A perfusionist must obtain a bachelor's degree that includes specific science and math requirements before applying to one of approximately 18 postgraduate programs across the country. Most programs include 12 months of didactic learning followed by 12 months of clinical training. Some programs grant a certificate and others award a master's degree. After successful completion of an accredited program, a graduate must perform a prescribed number of independent procedures before applying to take scientific and clinical exams. Upon passing both exams, the distinction of Certified Clinical Perfusionist (CCP) is awarded.

■ PRIMARY ROLE

The perfusionist's primary role is the setup and operation of the cardiopulmonary bypass (CPB) system, also known as extracorporeal circulation (ECC) (Figure 4.18). The purpose of CPB is to divert the flow of blood away from the heart and lungs so that the cardiac surgeon can work on a still or non-beating heart. Some of the procedures that require the use of CPB are coronary artery bypass grafts, heart valve repair or replacement, repair of aortic dissection or aneurysm, repair of congenital heart defects, trauma, and heart or lung transplantation. Other OR activities for a perfusionist may include assisting with blood salvage techniques, platelet gel processing for wound healing, anticoagulation monitoring, bypass for liver transplantation, and the administration of hyperthermic chemotherapy to specific areas of the body.

Additional cardiopulmonary therapies that a perfusionist can be involved with—often outside of the OR—include intraaortic balloon initiation and monitoring, extracorporeal membrane oxygenation setup and monitoring, and ventricular assist device support.

When a patient is on CPB, the perfusionist is expected to meet the patient's metabolic needs and preserve organ function. In order to do this, the perfusionist needs to pay particular attention to the patient's mean arterial pressure and blood flow (based on body surface area), urine output, and cerebral oximetry. Adequate blood electrolyte and red cell concentration, and appropriate anticoagulation status must also be monitored.

In order to provide optimal patient care, the perfusionist works closely with the surgeon, anesthesiologist, and nursing team (Figure 4.19). The language used

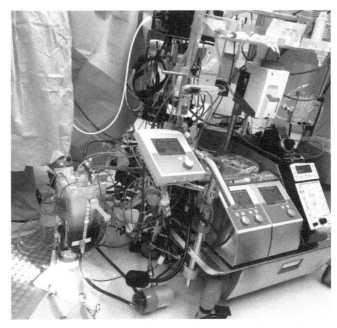

FIGURE 4.18 The bypass machine is one of the most fascinating machines in the operating room to see at work, but is also a dangerous trip hazard. Be mindful of it as you back away from the table or move about the OR. (Photo used with permission from Jennie O'Shea, University of Utah.)

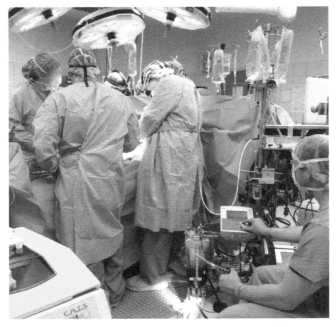

FIGURE 4.19 The perfusionist (seated) is in constant communication with the surgeon. (Photo used with permission from Jennie O'Shea, University of Utah.)

can be very specific to a cardiac operating room and allows the team to work safely and efficiently together. With time and experience, a new practitioner will understand the meaning and importance of these phrases and cue words.

Perfusionists, like other members of the OR team, are one specialized part of that team, and we are here to provide optimal patient care and assist new and seasoned practitioners with the knowledge they need to progress and provide the best patient care possible. We often do that quietly, almost inconspicuously, but with great vigilance; many patients and practitioners are completely unaware of our presence.

CHAPTER 5

Teamwork and Communication in the Operating Room

• *Louise Hull, PhD and Nick Sevdalis, PhD*

There is something captivating about witnessing an operating room (OR) team perform as a "team" to accomplish what is, to many people, the extraordinary: invasive procedures to the human body that cure disease (Figure 5.1). In contrast, there is an amazing sense of exasperation witnessing a team work as disconnected (and sometimes competing) individuals to try and accomplish what only a team can accomplish. If you haven't done so already, you will experience both the captivation and exasperation of OR teamwork; hopefully more of the former, but prepare yourself for the latter.

If you have never witnessed the triumphs and failures of OR teamwork, you may be questioning why teamwork and communication in the OR are important enough to warrant a chapter dedicated to them. This is a fair question and one that we have been asked many times over the years. For the past 10–15 years, researchers around the world have spent countless hours conducting observational studies exploring the quality of communication and teamwork in the OR. The findings do not paint a pretty picture—communication and teamwork failures occur frequently, causing not only tension in the OR but also compromising patient safety.

To try to improve this state of affairs, comparisons have been made with other industries to highlight the importance of teamwork and communication in the OR. Perhaps the most common—and the most irritating to OR teams—is comparison to the aviation industry. There are so many obvious differences between surgical patients and modern aircraft that we do not need to highlight them here. There is, however, an important similarity between the two industries: strong evidence exists that serious mishaps in aviation (plane crashes) and in the OR (the patient dies or is seriously harmed in the course of an operation) are frequently associated with breakdowns in communication and teamwork. Many of the important

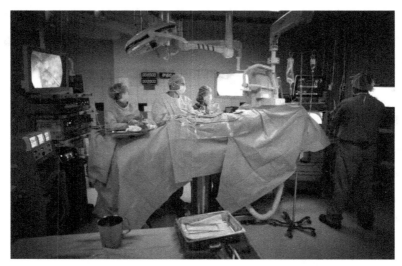

FIGURE 5.1 It takes a full team to care for a patient in the OR. (Photo used with permission from Charlie Ehlert, University of Utah.)

lessons that the aviation industry has learned from analyzing accidents have been adopted by the surgical community to improve the safety and quality of surgical care—the use of checklists is perhaps one of the most prominent ones.

In what follows, we highlight the uniqueness of OR teams, throw in a few anecdotes from the many hours (weeks, months, and years) we have spent being a "fly on the wall" in the OR, as well as a bit of scientific evidence—as we all love evidence-based medicine and practice—to help you appreciate the importance of communication and teamwork in the OR.

It is easy for an OR newbie to jump to the Orwellian conclusion that although the OR consists of a team, some members of the team are "more equal" than others. Both authors of this chapter initially believed this, and we think this has a lot to do with the different personalities and egos in the OR. Trust us, it will not take you long to realize this is not the case. As a thought experiment, let's consider the ability of the OR team to accomplish the end goal (safe, high quality surgery) minus one member of the team. For good measure, let's consider three scenarios:

1. No anesthesiologist: The patient would be awake. In essence, the OR team would be transported back to the time before anesthetics (i.e., the nineteenth century) when surgery was a painful, traumatic, and horrific experience for patients (and likely many of those involved in performing the surgery).
2. No surgeon: The patient would have a nice deep sleep (facilitated by the person at the top end of the table) but would wake up with the same problem that brought them to the OR in the first place. The scrub technician, the circulating nurses, and everyone else in OR would have beautifully prepared the OR in anticipation for the operation, but without the surgeons they soon would be very bored, with nothing to do.

3. No scrub technician: The patient would be asleep, but the surgeon would have no instruments to operate—or at the very least they would have to sort out everything themselves ahead of every procedure, thus limiting their ability to do as many procedures.

What we hope this experiment demonstrates is that every member of the OR team is critical—surgery is a team sport, and its goals cannot be accomplished without the entire team pulling together. The mini-scenarios above are extreme and hopefully unrealistic to highlight the point [although we have been in the OR many a time when no one seems to know where the surgeon(s) have disappeared to], but it is important to appreciate the unique but complementary knowledge, skills, roles, and responsibilities that each member of the OR team brings to the table. It also leads to the next important point: the OR team is a group of well-educated, extensively trained professionals, who when brought together are much more than the sum of its individual parts.

Another point to consider in relation to communication and teamwork in the OR is that these skills are not as strongly associated with surgical expertise as technical and psychomotor skills. This means you may have senior surgeons or anesthesiologists in the OR with little in the way of good communication skills.

Here is an amusing episode from the experience of one of us in the OR. One day, after introducing ourselves as patient safety scientists conducting team observations, the attending surgeon retorted "I define my expertise in terms of my technical ability, not my ability to work as a team." (Fair comment, especially considering that until recently the outcome of an operation was thought to be the function of two things: first, how sick the patient is and second, how technically gifted and skilled the operating surgeon is.) Before we had a chance to consider this statement position, the surgeon quickly followed up with a challenge: "If you can prove to me that my teamwork has an impact on my technical ability then you'll have my attention." The gauntlet had been thrown down. So we did what any academic would do: we trundled back to the comfort of our office and spent some time contemplating how best to scientifically approach this challenge. We gathered evidence via a systematic review of the literature that revealed a clear picture: better teamwork is associated with better technical performance (an oversimplification of the results, but this is the bottom line finding). We are not sure whether the surgeon in question ever read this work but the bottom line finding remains, and it gets stronger every day. Fast forward to the present day, and you'll find that the evidence is mounting that better teamwork is associated with not only better technical performance on the part of the surgeon, but also with decreased morbidity and mortality rates. (If you are not convinced, a PubMed search will do the trick: research groups around the world have contributed to the proof.) Perhaps the most important point that you should take away from reading this chapter is to never underestimate the power and importance of effective teamwork.

Let's leave ORs aside for a moment. In many ways, the OR team is similar to the functional and dysfunctional teams that we have all been part of throughout our lives outside the OR. The degree of functionality/dysfunctionality will vary, and there will always be individuals with whom you will work well and individuals with whom you will struggle to work well. Being a conscientious and well-rounded professional means that you need to be able to work safely and effectively even with people you have not chosen to be on the same team with—the overriding concern is always the safety and wellbeing of the patient on the table, who has entrusted their life to the team's hands.

Just like other skills, good communication and good teamwork come more naturally to some than to others. Some people are seen as "good communicators," just like some of us have better psychomotor dexterity. Still, no one would dream of taking on a surgical procedure before completing years of education and training, and the same applies to team and communication skills. Training is needed in these skills as well. With good training you will perfect these skills over time. As an OR newbie, you and your patients are lucky, as you have entered the world of surgery at an exciting time: simulation-based training is now a permanent fixture in most training programs. You will no doubt experience the fun, sweat, and terror of simulation. You will learn how to deal with "difficult" team members and how to cope in the crisis situations you will face. The military adage, "train hard, fight easy" is relevant here. Training makes you better prepared to face tough crises—even those rare ones that you may or may not face in a lifetime of surgical practice. The last thing you want is to face a crisis without ever having rehearsed it.

We have been in the OR when things have gone dramatically wrong. It wasn't until we experienced the terror of facing the reality that the patient on the table might die in front of our eyes that we really appreciated how important effective communication and teamwork in the OR is. It's not until you see a team facing this situation pull together to turn the situation around that you really appreciate the role that each member of the team can play in a high-functioning OR. Every member of the OR team, regardless of seniority and role, has the potential to get you out of a sticky situation or prevent you from experiencing one. This is the true glory of effective teamwork—there will be always be someone, perhaps the person you least expect, to dig you out of a hole—for example, a medical student who questions the attending surgeon about whether the surgeon is operating on the correct side, preventing wrong-site surgery. Anyone on the team should feel part of that team, and can prevent a disaster from happening.

So, newbies, enjoy the complex environment that is the OR. You will learn a lot in it and you will contribute to patient care. Whenever you step into an OR, remember the importance of effective communication and teamwork.

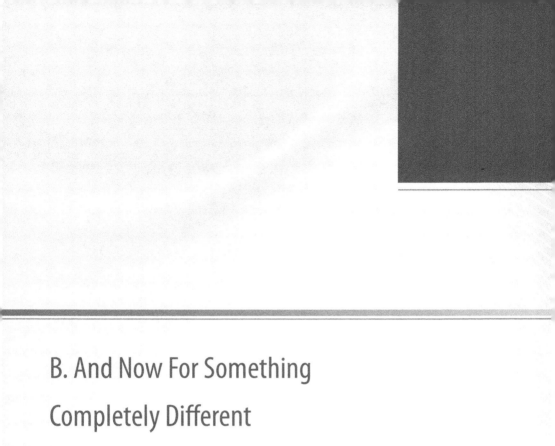

B. And Now For Something Completely Different

CHAPTER 6

The OR and Humor

• *Ruth Braga, MSN, RN*

I used to be a very well mannered individual. Then two things happened:

1. I went to nursing school.
2. I got a job in a Level I trauma center OR.

Somehow, during the course of those two things, the filter that every "normal" individual has auto-installed in the brain began to disappear. It still worked, but sometimes the reaction was significantly delayed. I noticed an increased frequency of my mouth running ahead of my brain, and I was cracking jokes that I would have never cracked in my former life.

I also noticed that I wasn't alone. Many of the surgeons and anesthesia staff I worked with also lacked this filter. I worked in various operating rooms in the United States and figured the humor would vary based on geographic location.

It didn't.

Whether it is a small private surgical center or a large Level I trauma teaching institution, the operating room is a glorious melting pot of individuals who have been trained all over the world. Surgeons, anesthesia, residents, staff, students, and others come from a variety of institutions. Each has their own way of handling the stress that they deal with.

I have often heard nursing and medical students comment on the fact that what is said in the OR is irreverent and not funny. Some are turned off from working in the OR because of our odd sense of humor, lack of filter, and apparent inability to demonstrate humane levels of sensitivity.

Why do we do this? Are we just horrible people? It wasn't just staff—I'd cared for cancer patients who joked about being bald, and a fresh amputee who laughed about being "down a limb." What was wrong with these people?

To make sure I hadn't entirely lost the sensitive side of myself, I did some research. Not only is this humor found in environments such as operating rooms, emergency rooms, and intensive care units, it has also been used by patients, and it has a name: *gallows humor.* Wikipedia defines it as "witticism in the face of—and in response to—a hopeless situation. It arises from stressful, traumatic, or life-threatening situations, often in circumstances such that death is perceived as impending and unavoidable." It seems that someone at some point in history cracked a joke shortly before being hanged, and the term stuck. Why would this matter in the trauma operating room?

The next time you visit the OR, take a moment to think about the bigger picture and see how the above definition of gallows humor might fit in.

A group of individuals gathers in a room filled with intimidating technology, extreme temperatures, and multiple personal hazards. It may be the second or two-hundredth time that they have worked together—their experience ranges from months to decades. Each is hoping that they have the skill and knowledge needed—not necessarily for this procedure, but for what this particular surgeon, anesthesiologist, nurse, scrub technician, and others will need—in order to get the job done.

An almost-naked patient is wheeled into the room. Only a few know the patient's history. The rest are only aware of what brought them to the OR that day. The ability to move about freely becomes limited as blue drapes turn every-thing within a two-foot radius of the patient into what is universally known as the "touch-and-die" zone. For the next few minutes to hours, each person will care-fully and craftily dodge, duck, and maneuver their way around this room.

For hours, they stand shoulder to shoulder under hot, bright lights. Hands work in tiny spaces. Items are constantly counted. Each individual fights the instinct to be repulsed by what surrounds them. The urge to eat, drink, sleep, and visit the bathroom is suppressed, or quickly addressed. Teaching is intense, and there is no ducking out or changing the subject if you don't know the answer. Restart buttons don't exist.

If you are wondering how you could you possibly laugh or make jokes in this setting, I will assure you that humor is a coping mechanism here. Although we are surrounded by high stress, tragedy, loss, and at times impending death, our ability to laugh with one another bonds us, gets us through, and keeps us coming back. Sometimes we take it for granted that we work behind the red line, away from the public and patients who are awake. We *do* need to be mindful of the fact that we are often cloistered, and gallows humor is certainly not an excuse for a tasteless verbal free-for-all.

The next time you hear a surgeon, nurse or anesthesiologist make a joke about the mismatched socks on the pair of dismembered legs accompanying the man run over by a train, refer to a toddler who fell out a third story window as "failure to fly," or laugh hysterically at the fact that someone was shot right in the center of their gun tattoo, we hope you will remember (and appreciate) the value and purpose of our sense of humor.

Personalities in the Operating Room

• *Ross M. Blagg, MD*

Analogies make it easier for all of us normal folks to relate to complex things. For instance, if you are a surgical resident, the operating room (OR) will be like your football stadium. You will experience triumphs and severe defeats but in the end, hopefully you will nail the Super Bowl and end up being the bomb.com when it comes to surgery.

Maybe the closest you have ever come to the operating room is watching *Grey's Anatomy*. While that steamy drama offers some nice couch entertainment, the real deal is a little different, and you probably won't run into Meredith Grey or Dr. McSteamy. If you are about to dive into this operative world, you are going to want to have a few pearls up your scrub sleeves. My chosen analogy for the OR is to think of it as the ocean. Now, the ocean can be a really scary place if we go all *Jaws* with the comparison, or it can be more pleasant, like *Finding Nemo*. The point is, much like the ocean, the OR can be a fantastical world full of intrigue and positive messages such as "keep on swimming," or it can be the place of your blood-in-the-water demise. Yikes! That's dramatic. Either way, let's get to know your operating neighbors.

■ THE SCRUB SINK

This will be your first stop on your way into the OR. I like to think of the scrub sink as the tiny shrimp on the ocean floor. If you just patiently place your hands on the sandy bottom while diving in the ocean, these little guys and gals will scurry out of their holes and start cleaning your fingernails. A few things to know about the sink: it will likely either be motion- or foot pedal-activated (no knobs to turn) (Figure 7.1). If you have never scrubbed in before, ask someone to walk you through the process. It can seem a little awkward the first few times. The great thing about the sink is that it won't yell or make fun of you. And if you mess up your first try at scrubbing, you simply start again. Just keep swimming…

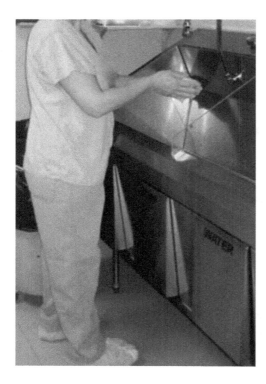

FIGURE 7.1 At the scrub sink. This model requires the use of your knee to turn the water on or off. (Photo used with permission from Ruth Braga, University of Utah.)

■ THE CIRCULATOR/OR NURSE

The circulator nurse is like a sailfish (extremely fast). This person darts around making sure the room is appropriately stocked with whatever is needed to make the surgical case go swiftly and smoothly. Many of these guys/gals have been around since before you were in diapers, and this means she/he knows more than you. You should know that before walking into the room. Always respect their space and their time because they are very busy and will be darting from the computer to the shelves to the OR table like a sailfish on Adderall. Be sure to introduce yourself to the circulator before scrubbing in and write your name on the whiteboard in the room (Figure 7.2) so that the circulator knows who you are. Always offer to grab your own gown and gloves off the shelf to hand to the scrub tech (see below). But remember that if you've not done this before, ask for help so that you can maintain sterility.

■ THE SCRUB TECHNICIAN (SCRUB TECH)

The scrub tech is like a clownfish (Nemo) and the "scrub table" is the sea anemone. The tech never gets too far from the anemone. Remember to never touch the table, because just like an anemone, it will sting you, and you will likely upset the clownfish. The scrub tech passes instruments to and from the surgeon. Often this

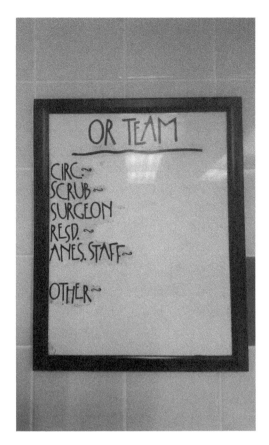

FIGURE 7.2 Write your name and glove size on the white board in the OR. (Photo used with permission from Ruth Braga, University of Utah.)

will be a very quick and efficient process with instruments flying off the table and into hands with crazy speed. You, my newbie, will want to stand clear. Remember, nobody likes the middleman, so don't try to be him. While it can seem helpful to pass the instruments from the scrub tech to the surgeon, this is not necessary or wanted. If you see the scrub tech holding an instrument out, waiting for the surgeon to grab it, just let it be. The surgeon will take it herself when she is ready (Figure 7.3).

■ THE ANESTHESIOLOGIST

The anesthesiologist is like a lobster hanging out in the crevices of a coral reef, sometimes a little hidden, but really important to the life cycle. When you are new to the OR, the anesthesiologist can be a good friend to have, especially before you scrub into the case. Prior to getting sterile, there is a lot that happens in the room, including putting the patient to sleep and placing a breathing tube. Hang out with the lobster and you're likely to see some cool stuff before the surgery ever begins. And remember, when making requests of the anesthesiologist during the case,

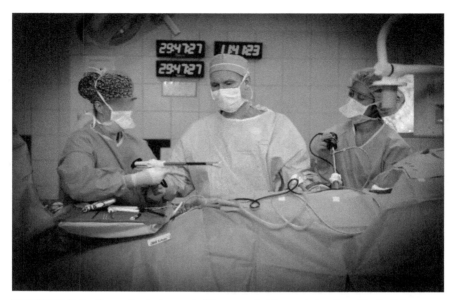

FIGURE 7.3 Patiently passing instruments. (Photo used with permission from Charlie Ehlert, University of Utah.)

such as having him/her move the IV pole so you can squeeze closer to the surgical site, always use your "please" and "thank you" nice words. All lobsters appreciate this.

■ THE PATIENT

The patient is the whale shark—that big slumbering creature that will sometimes pass by the reef. He just minds his own business, mouth open, feeding on plankton. Remember that patients are at their most vulnerable state in the OR because they are under general anesthesia. So don't rest your elbow on the whale shark's head. The patient should always be your number one priority. If you remember this at all times and make all decisions based on that principle, you will be okay. So when you contaminate yourself by touching something that isn't draped in blue (blue drapes indicate sterility), always speak up and change out those gloves and/ or that gown. You may feel a little ridiculous, but remember that we have all done it, and not saying anything will be putting that whale shark in danger. Keep on swimming, little buddy.

■ THE SURGEON

This is the shark. Before you get your undies all bunched up, remember that sharks come in many varieties. Maybe you'll get lucky for your first OR go-around and end up with a nurse shark. But it's best to be prepared for the gummy, rows-of-teeth, *Carcharodon carcharias* (a.k.a. the Great White).

Step one is to know some anatomy. This is a fairly easy exercise. For instance, if you are going to be operating on the abdomen, then take a look at the anatomy of the abdomen the night before the case. Memorize things such as the layers of the abdominal wall and where the intestines live in relation to other abdominal organs. If you are going to be operating on a foot, look up the muscles of the foot and what vessels supply the foot, and where the vessels and nerves exist in relation to the foot. For the most part, if you know some anatomy, most surgeons will be pretty pleased and will involve you in the procedure, which is much more fun that just standing there.

Now, if you're looking for honors, then it's important to remember that sharks can be pretty full of themselves. Even the nice, smiling ones have worked really hard to achieve and maintain their oceanic position, so a little recognition never hurts. You can easily Google and/or PubMed search your shark's name to find any articles he/she has written. If any of the articles pertain to your own interests or to the procedure being performed, read it, and then mention it when it seems relevant. The ensuing conversation might be the ticket to making you feel right at home in the operating room.

◼ YOU

"Me?" you might ask. Yes, you. You, too, are now a part of this operating room. You are the remora fish (sometimes called a suckerfish) that latches onto the shark and goes on those shark journeys throughout the hospital. This is such a great position to be in because you get to have fairly little responsibility and you get to glean all you can from your surroundings. Take advantage of the view. If you have a question, ask. If you don't understand something, ask. Just make sure you are nice about it. You know, use those nice people words like "please" and "thanks." Also, mind your mouth just a little. Don't be too chatty and don't get too casual, even if those around you seem to be letting loose a bit. Similar to observing sharks and other sea creatures from a safe distance, remember to be professional and to keep a safe "distance" in the OR. Overall, a good remora is observant. Look around for ways you might be helpful. You may think you have no skills to offer, but you do have legs and arms. Before the surgery even starts, the patient needs help getting onto the surgical table and the patient's bed needs to be wheeled out into the hallway. It's always appreciated when you help with this. Similarly, when the case is over, help get the patient off the table and onto the bed. Watch your resident for other ways you might assist.

◼ THE RESIDENT

Imagine a remora fish that is a little bit bigger than you and wears glasses—that's the surgical resident. This remora is your partner. You are both latched onto the shark. He or she is a little more experienced and wiser than you, and you should use this to your advantage. Follow your resident's lead and direct most of your questions to your resident. Importantly, never try to make your resident look bad or act as though you know more than the resident. For instance, if the resident is

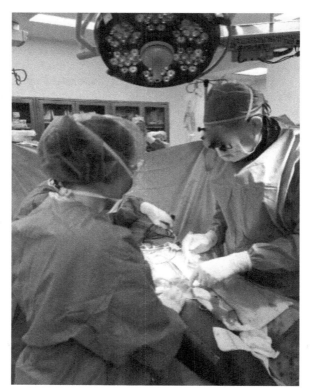

FIGURE 7.4 Watch, listen, learn and enjoy. (Photo used with permission from Sarah Bryczkowski, Rutgers New Jersey Medical School.)

asked a question and seems to be stumped, don't jump in because you know the answer. Wait until you are asked to do so. The surgeon will not respect you for one-upping, and your resident remora might swim away, leaving you all alone in the deep blue ocean (Figure 7.4).

Well, it's time to get excited. Having reviewed the crew that lies within the deep blue waters, you've essentially stuck in your big toe to test out the temperature. Now all that's left is for you to cannonball right on in. Enjoy the swim.

2015 Grammy Awards Category: Music in the Operating Room

• *Winner: Marie Crandall, MD, MPH, FACS*

It has been two years since the publication of the seminal article, "Surgeon Preference and Music in the Operating Room: A Randomized, Controlled Trial" by Crandall et al.[1] A highly regarded[2] and frequently cited[3] study, it highlighted the importance of musical choice in the operating room. Key findings included unanimous agreement that when a patient is critically injured or ill, music is a distraction and should be off or very low; however, nearly all surgeons were comfortable with music during less urgent procedures.

As noted in the Crandall study, nearly all work examining music in the OR has been patient-focused in terms of intraoperative and postoperative comfort, analgesic needs, and anesthetic requirements. Subsequent to this, a systematic review and meta-analysis was published in *The Lancet*, which concluded that music in nearly every form, irrespective of timing, duration, or musical choice, helped reduce postoperative pain and narcotic needs.[4] As the 2015 Grammy Award Winner for Music in the Operating Room, I need to declare this conclusion both deeply disturbing and potentially dangerous. The idea that the choice of music is irrelevant to patient outcomes has clearly never been studied in an operating room with a surgeon playing only show tunes for 12 hours. The same 12 songs OVER and OVER and OVER. It's even worse if it's from a children's movie. How can that not make your eyes water and hands shake? All of the authors (MC), and I imagine many readers, would agree that these musical choices could not help but contribute to postoperative wound infections and hemorrhoids.

Happily, I have been an attending for over a decade, so I am no longer subject to the kind of suffering I once endured. But I do vividly remember the days of endless re-do liver transplants and Whipples with portal venous reconstructions and the assaults on my sensibilities from endless operettas and Modest Mouse marathons.

Please, as a courtesy to your trainees, treat intraoperative musical choice with the same kind of measured respect and attention to the literature that you would, say, preoperative cardiac evaluations. We surgeons are frequently, some would say inherently, narcissistic, so we do not consider the effect of our music on our trainees, the OR staff, and anesthesiologists. That is simply villainous. Think what would happen if we had no control at all and the music were piped in overhead after being carefully selected by The Joint Commission. If we continue to be serial offenders, afflicting our colleagues with Justin Bieber or Celine Dion, we will see a revolt and it will soon be out of our hands.

Because I think it is important to be solution-focused, not simply problem-focused, and I do not take the title of 2015 Grammy Award Winner for Music in the Operating Room lightly, I have devised a philanthropic strategy to address the distressingly terrible music in the OR, which could lead to boils and plagues of grasshoppers. If you post/link/Tweet this reference (@vegansurgeon), I will send you a playlist of either 15 or 30 songs (see Appendix for a sample) that should get you through most normal OR days. It will include everything except opera, modern country, techno, and most popular vocalists after the year 1999. I don't use playlists myself because I prefer to go alphabetically song by song down the 6000 songs on my phone, but not everyone has that luxury.

Now, to be sure, Spotify or Pandora are also reasonable choices, but with those services you run the risk of advertisements and the sheer terror of a really dreadful song coming on at a crucial moment, which then may lead to death or dismemberment.[5]

■ APPENDIX

Sample 15-song playlist:

1. *El Shing-a-Ling*, Poncho Sanchez
2. *Keep it Comin' Love*, KC and the Sunshine Band
3. *Baba O'Riley*, The Who
4. *East St. Louis Toodle-O*, Duke Ellington
5. *Walk on By*, Dionne Warwick
6. *Sabotage*, Beastie Boys
7. *P. Funk*, Parliament
8. *Fairies Wear Boots*, Black Sabbath
9. *Radar Love*, Golden Earring
10. *Rebel Girl*, Bikini Kill
11. *Yesterday Once More*, The Carpenters
12. *Da Mystery of Chessboxin'*, Wu-Tang Clan
13. *Mob Clash*, The Effigies
14. *Hang on to Your Love*, Sade
15. *California Love*, 2Pac feat. Dr. Dre

Have fun out there and be safe. Don't let The Joint Commission bring us down and ruin our ambiance in the OR.[6]

■ REFERENCES

1. Crandall M AWS Blog. https://www.womensurgeons.org/surgeon-preference-and-music-in-the-operating-room-a-randomized-controlled-trial/.
2. All of my friends liked it and said it was funny.
3. I personally Tweeted and retweeted it at least twice.
4. Hole J, Hirsch M, Ball E, Meads C. Music as an aid for postoperative recovery in adults: a systematic review and meta-analysis. *The Lancet* 2015;386(10004): 1659–1671.
5. The authors would like to note that people are shot and dismembered every day for their musical choices. And then buried with broken CDs of One Direction and Michael Bolton.
6. The authors (MC) would like to acknowledge the willing and capable assistance of University of Florida Jacksonville surgery residents and SICU ARNPs who provided moral support and Dr. Raquel Weston who graciously read the first draft and politely laughed, though she did comment that she does like show tunes and the music of Disney movies.

Intraop (In the OR)

CHAPTER 9

Welcome to the Jungle: The Five Senses of the Operating Room

- *Elizabeth Hanes, BSN, RN*

If you parachuted into the Amazon jungle tomorrow, you might expect all of your senses to be stimulated by the new environment. Your nostrils would filter the pungent smell of leaves rotting on the jungle floor. Your eyes would take in colorful parrots darting between the trees. You might even "taste" the warm humidity of the air as you breathed it in.

The operating room is a lot like the jungle in that it stimulates all of your senses. From the moment you walk through the door of the OR, your five senses will kick into overdrive. Here's what to expect.

■ SIGHT

When you first enter the OR before the start of a case, you will see a whirlwind of activity (Figure 9.1). While there won't be any parrots in sight, you will see many people swooping from pre-op holding to supply room to operating suite, often carrying armloads of supplies and paperwork. You will score points with the circulating nurse if you offer to help carry some of this equipment, but be careful where you set it once inside the room. Don't touch or approach anything blue in color (Figure 9.2), because blue represents the sterile field.

The OR may be second only to the Amazon for richness of color. You won't be bedazzled by the gorgeous blooms of tropical flowers like you might in the jungle, but you will take in a variety of hues, including the blue of the gowns worn by surgeons, residents, and scrub techs, the gleaming silver of stainless steel instruments, the red of blood spilling from the surgeon's incisions, and the pink, yellow, and white of tissues inside the body (Figure 9.3). In terms of the visual experience of

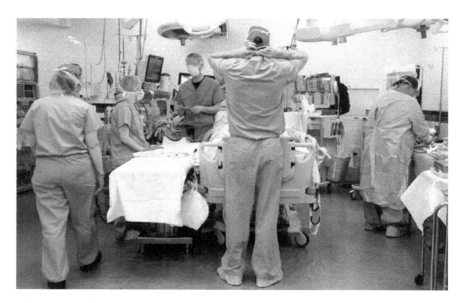

FIGURE 9.1 The burn team gets ready to move a patient to the OR table. Note the scrub techni-cian working to set up his table, anesthesiology at the head of the bed, and plenty of hands to help move the patient to the OR table. (Photo used with permission from Ruth Braga, University of Utah.)

the OR, seeing the inside of a person's body is perhaps the most fascinating aspect of this setting. Visualizing a beating heart marks a profound moment inside any OR, no matter how many times you've seen it. Your sight contributes a great deal to the richness of the OR experience (Figure 9.4).

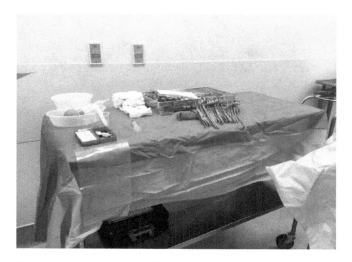

FIGURE 9.2 Back-table setup for a case at UCLA's Breast Center. (Photo used with permission from Deanna Attai, UCLA.)

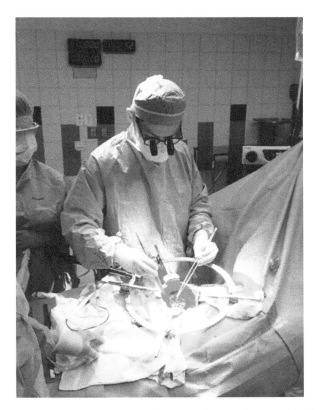

FIGURE 9.3 The Bookwalter retractor during a kidney transplant case. (Photo used with permission from the University of Utah Transplant Team.)

■ SMELL

What the eyes giveth, the nose may taketh away. In the jungle, the lush green of the flora may look breathtaking, but the stench of rotting plant material might leave you breathless for a moment. The OR is no different in this respect. Smell may be the most visceral of all senses, evoking responses ranging from nostalgic to nauseating. Before you enter the OR, prepare yourself for the myriad new odors you'll be encountering.

The electrocautery device (often called by the brand name "Bovie") burns human tissue to stop it from bleeding. When the surgeon employs this device your eyes may register innocuous gray-white smoke rising from the surgical field, but your nose will inhale the acrid odor only burning human flesh can produce. You may find the smell disgusting or nauseating at first but if you stay in the OR environment long enough, you soon will not give electrocautery smells a second thought (Figure 9.5).

Of all the unpleasant odors that can occur during surgery, one of the most horrific must be that of dead tissue, especially in the abdominal cavity. It's an unpleasant moment when the surgeon's knife pierces a distended belly and the smell of

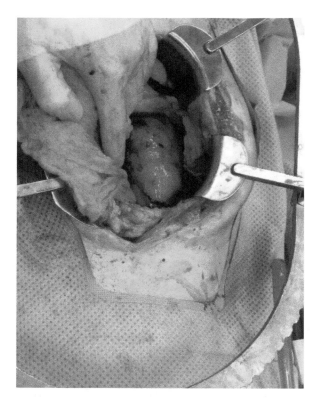

FIGURE 9.4 Transplanted kidney. (Photo used with permission from the University of Utah Transplant Team.)

necrotic bowel escapes into the air of the OR. Even seasoned nurses and doctors may retch and turn away. In anticipation of this possibility, many operating room personnel smear pungent ointment like mentholated petroleum jelly above their lip or inside their surgical mask prior to a potentially smelly case. If your nostrils are filled with the strong smell of menthol it's hard for your olfactory system to simultaneously process the purulent odor of gangrene.

Luckily you are more likely to notice the scent of the antiseptics used to clean the OR than to be subjected to a particularly foul-smelling case. And while the aroma of electrocautery abounds, it need not take you by surprise. The buzz of the instrument actuating will prepare you for the smell to follow.

■ SOUNDS

The jungle is never silent. Monkeys howl from the treetops, cicadas buzz in the canopy, and water trickles over rocks. Likewise, the operating room generates a constant hum from equipment and people. Some ORs may be quieter than others, but every operating room gives your hearing a workout.

As a surgical case gets underway, the environment can be very noisy. People might be dragging large pieces of equipment into the room. Monitors will emanate

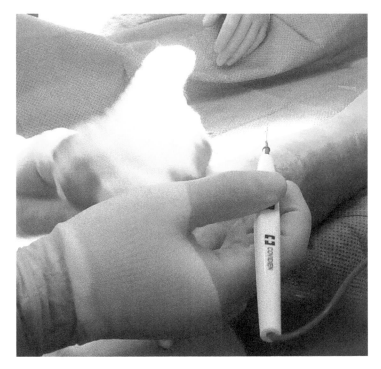

FIGURE 9.5 Bovie electrocautery "pencil" in hand to control bleeding. (Photo used with permission from Ruth Braga, University of Utah.)

their characteristic beeping sounds. Alarms may clang. Voices are often raised over the din of activity as everything is put into place.

Once the patient enters the room things usually quiet down significantly so the patient doesn't worry they might be interrupting a party. The noise level of a surgical suite often hews to the surgeon's preference. If the surgeon likes it quiet for concentration purposes or if something critical is occurring during a case, there will be very little background noise. If the surgeon has a more boisterous personality, then you may find the music turned up loud and the personnel chatting and laughing almost as raucously as howler monkeys. Often for routine cases you'll find that the OR noise levels are somewhere in the middle, though they can change quickly.

■ TOUCH

As you walk through the jungle, you'll feel soft grass beneath your feet. You'll brush away branches with your hand. You may even grip a heavy machete to chop away vines. Likewise, in the OR everyone uses their sense of touch to some degree, depending on their role.

The circulating nurse feels the stiff smoothness of sterile gown tags as she assists surgeons and residents into them. The nurse also holds packages that crackle, like suture packets, and bundles soft as a bunny, such as sterile trays in blue wrapping.

Because the circulator passes materials to the sterile field, he or she may handle warm instruments fresh from the sterilizer or cool syringes filled with liquid.

Of all the tactile sensations one may experience in the OR, the most important is that of the warm, reassuring hand on the patient's shoulder or arm as the patient drifts off to sleep. Nothing beats that skin-to-skin contact.

Surgeons, residents, and scrub technicians experience a different kind of human touch: they actually handle tissues and organs inside the body. Feeling adipose (fatty) tissue between your fingers or touching someone's lung creates sensations that are difficult to describe.

Of course, anyone within the sterile field also senses a heat that may rival a jungle's environment. Swathed in layers of clothing and toiling under bright, hot lights, the surgical team can begin to feel steamy quickly. For this reason many ORs set the thermostat very low, which can make those standing outside the field feel chilly. In ORs designated for burn or trauma or for pediatric patients, the thermostat may be set very warm to help the patient maintain their temperature. Yes, the operating room involves more tactile sensations than you might imagine (Figure 9.6).

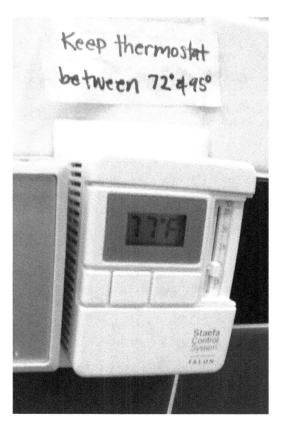

FIGURE 9.6 Thermostat in a burn OR. Burn ORs tend to be extremely warm because the patients have trouble controlling their temperature. (Photo used with permission from Ruth Braga, University of Utah.)

■ TASTE

In the jungle you might taste bitter berries or imbibe sweet coconut milk, but here the OR differs greatly from its Amazonian counterpart. Taste is perhaps the least-used sense in the operating room, because it is not a place for dining or drinking. No one should be chewing gum or sucking on a hard candy while in the OR, including those circulating outside the sterile field. We don't need something like the famous *Seinfeld* episode with the Junior Mint to happen!

Nonetheless, the smoke caused by electrocautery can indeed evoke a taste sensation. It is not unlike the taste of secondhand smoke, except the tang of electrocautery is much more ash-flavored than cigarette smoke. Anyone who spends much time in the OR gets used to the taste of electrocautery fast.

If thirst can be considered a "taste," then you likely will experience it. Those who stand gloved and gowned under the hot lights of the sterile field can get thirsty quickly as they perspire. Some people may also experience dry mouth during a procedure, whether due to dehydration or a fight-or-flight stress response triggered by something like the scent of gangrene.

It may not resemble the Amazon rain forest, but the operating room can feel like a jungle to newbies. Engage all five of your senses to fully experience this wonderful environment—and rest assured you'll live to tell about your new adventure.

CHAPTER 10

Robots and Ring Stands

Operating Room Equipment From A To Z

- *Diane Tyler, MSN, RN and Ruth Braga, MSN, RN*

When stepping into an operating room, you are entering an area of machines and equipment. Most ORs have the same standard equipment, but this can vary depending on the surgery that will take place. Each OR is staffed with a team of people who know how to use the equipment and machines in the room.

While there may be some variation in how each institution refers to different pieces of equipment, we hope you will get a good idea of the general items you will find.

■ AIR

Regular air won't do for our patients in the operating room—premium gases are piped in through ceiling mounts (Figure 10.1). Air and oxygen are the two most common. Remember the colors: air is yellow (Figure 10.2) and oxygen is green.

■ ANESTHESIA CART (SUPPLY)

An anesthesia supply cart (Figure 10.3) holds many of the supplies needed for every surgery. A well-stocked cart keeps equipment, from syringes to intubating equipment, at the anesthesiologist's fingertips.

■ ANESTHESIA MACHINE

The anesthesiologist has the important role of keeping the patient asleep and keeping the patient's pain under control during the surgery. The anesthesia machine (Figure 10.4) is the mechanical workhorse of administering anesthesia during the surgery. The anesthesiologist uses it to keep the patient safe, sleeping, and comfortable during the surgery. The anesthesia machine gives breaths to the patient while it delivers the appropriate mixture of oxygen and anesthetic gas. Until it is time to reduce the medications and wake the patient at the end of the surgery, the anesthesia machine sends information to the anesthesiologist to interpret and use.

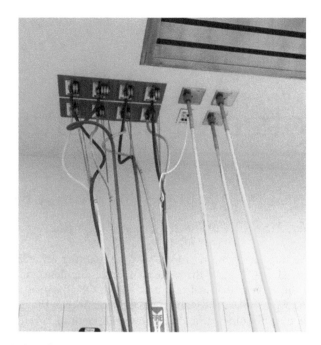

FIGURE 10.1 OR lines from the ceiling. (Photo used with permission from Diane Tyler, University of Utah.)

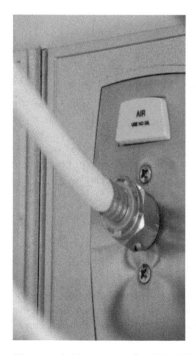

FIGURE 10.2 Air line up close. (Photo used with permission from Diane Tyler, University of Utah.)

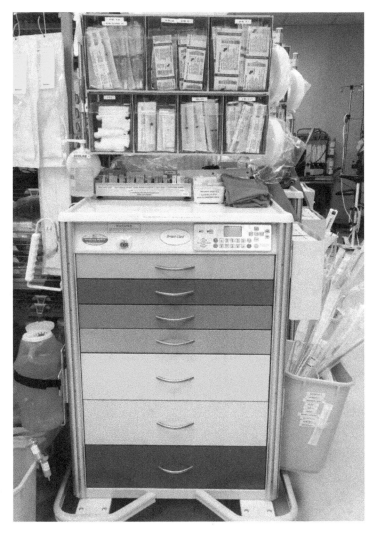

FIGURE 10.3 Fully stocked anesthesia cart. (Photo used with permission from Diane Tyler, University of Utah.)

Although the anesthesia machine looks complicated, it's really not that scary (Figure 10.5). The three canisters in the center are the different gases used to keep the patient asleep. The gauges provide information about oxygen and air delivery while the patient is having mechanical breaths given by the ventilator. The bellows mimics the movement of the lungs as it pushes air in and allows it to come back out. The anesthesia monitor displays important information about the patient's condition to the anesthesiologist during the entire surgical procedure (Figure 10.6).

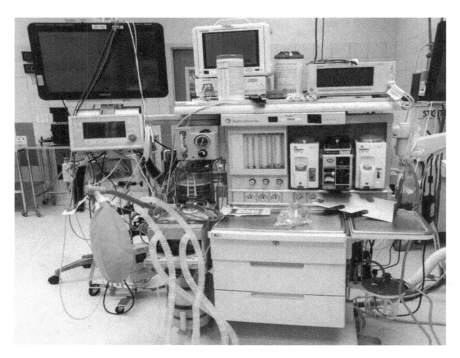

FIGURE 10.4 Anesthesia machine. (Photo used with permission from Diane Tyler, University of Utah.)

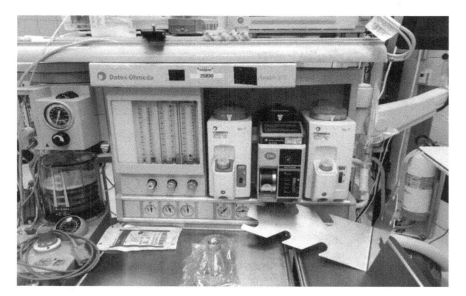

FIGURE 10.5 Anesthesia machine close-up. (Photo used with permission from Diane Tyler, University of Utah.)

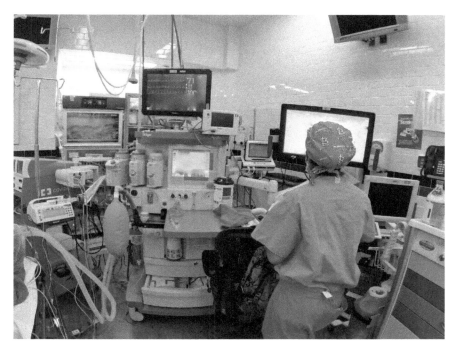

FIGURE 10.6 Anesthesia machine in use. (Photo used with permission from Ruth Braga, University of Utah.)

■ CLOCKS

In the OR, you will notice that we are obsessed with time (Figure 10.7). We note times of everything: in the room, to sleep, time out, when the incision is made, when the procedure ends, and when the patient leaves the room, just to name the most common ones. Counting or timing of almost any type, we can do it in the operating room.

■ CODE BUTTON

This is the last thing you want to be searching for when you need it. The code button (Figure 10.8) can be pushed to immediately notify other OR staff that a patient is arresting and help is needed right away. Thankfully, the place is filled with anesthesiologists and surgeons, and the ones who are available typically come running in herds when this button is pushed. You will have many OR-experienced hands to help out. When a code happens, your job is to do whatever you are told. Whether that is "MOVE!" or "HOLD THIS," help, watch, and learn, but always know where the button is.

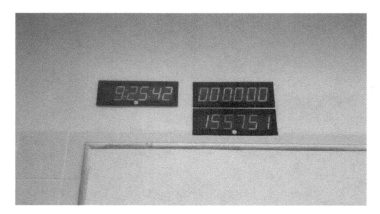

FIGURE 10.7 Clocks in the OR. (Photo used with permission from Ruth Braga, University of Utah.)

◼ ELECTRICAL/FLOOR BOXES

There is a tremendous amount of electricity used in the operating room, and outlets are everywhere. The outlet boxes are heavy grade and can be moved along the floor and hung from the ceiling (Figures 10.9 and 10.10). These floor boxes are like premeditated trip lines—be cautious.

◼ ELECTROCAUTERY (BOVIE)

This is an electrical cutting device that, when activated by the surgeon, cuts through skin and cauterizes vessels at the same time (Figure 10.11). It requires the use of a "Bovie pad" in order to work. This pad, which looks like a large blue

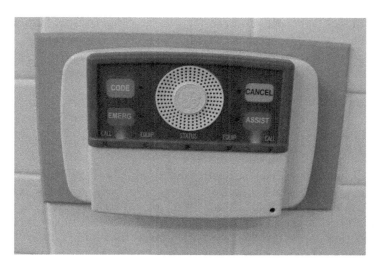

FIGURE 10.8 Code button in the OR. (Photo used with permission from Ruth Braga, University of Utah.)

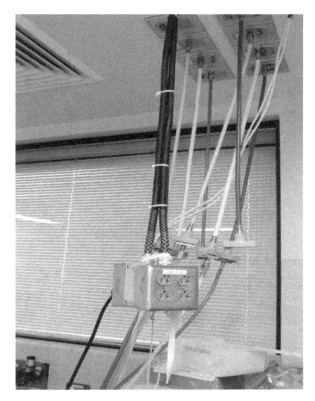

FIGURE 10.9 Ceiling lines in use. (Photo used with permission from Diane Tyler, University of Utah.)

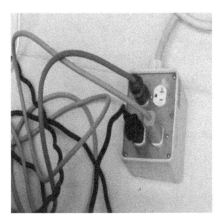

FIGURE 10.10 Floor electrical boxes. (Photo used with permission from Diane Tyler, University of Utah.)

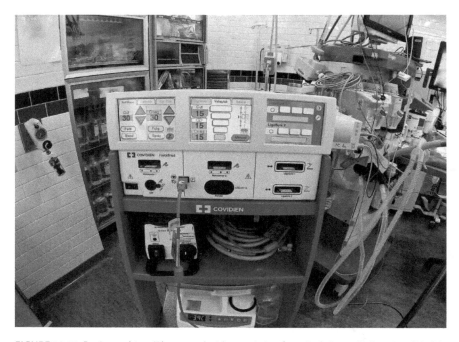

FIGURE 10.11 Bovie machine. (Photo used with permission from Ruth Braga, University of Utah.)

sticker, provides a ground for the electrical current that the Bovie sends through the patient's body. This sticker should go on a spot on the patient that is dry, hairless, free from injury, away from the operative site, and has a healthy amount of fatty tissue (usually the thigh, buttocks, bicep—whatever you can find that is "meaty"). Location of the grounding pad and skin condition when it is removed at the end of the surgical case should be documented.

■ GLOVES

Both sterile and non-sterile gloves are kept around the operating room (Figure 10.12). Non-sterile should be used for moving patients and other tasks around the operating room. Sterile gloves come in half sizes and are made of various materials, including latex-free if you are sensitive. If you can't find them, just ask. Double-gloving policies vary by institution—just remember that an additional layer of glove can provide one more barrier between you and getting stuck by a needle.

■ HEADLIGHTS

Even though the OR lights are bright, it can be helpful for surgeons to wear a headlight during cases where they are working in cavernous areas (Figure 10.13). The pinpoint direct light of a headlight provides better visibility. Ideally, the surgeon places the headlight on their head *before* scrubbing in, and the circulator plugs the

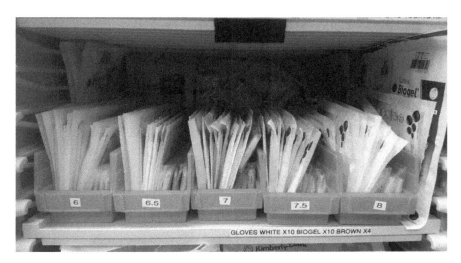

FIGURE 10.12 Various gloves. (Photo used with permission from Ruth Braga, University of Utah.)

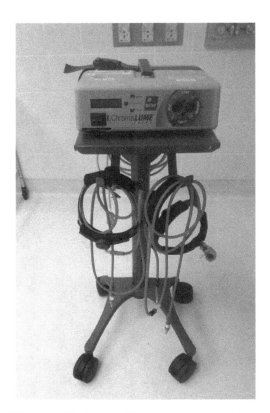

FIGURE 10.13 Headlight setup. (Photo used with permission from Ruth Braga, University of Utah.)

cord into the light box when the surgeon is gowned, gloved, and in their operative position. These present a special challenge if the surgeon decides to move and forgets that they are plugged in.

■ LIGHTS

The overhead OR lights are super-bright so the surgical field is flooded like a Friday night football game. The lights can be positioned to illuminate the surgical field, head to toe.

OR lights come in various styles, as do their controls (Figure 10.14 and 10.15). To ensure that the surgeon or others who are up at the field can maneuver them without contamination, handles are attached to the lights (Figure 10.16). When the surgeon, scrub technician, or resident are of varying heights, the handles may

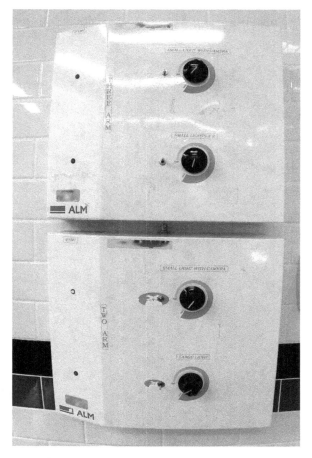

FIGURE 10.14 Controls for overhead OR lights. (Photo used with permission from Ruth Braga, University of Utah.)

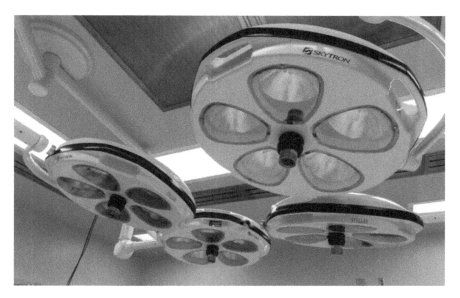

FIGURE 10.15 OR lights. (Photo used with permission from Ruth Braga, University of Utah.)

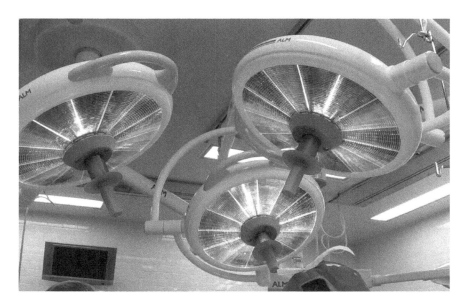

FIGURE 10.16 OR lights without sterile handles. (Photo used with permission from Ruth Braga, University of Utah.)

get bumped and contaminated. If you feel a bump against your head, speak up, because the handle needs to be changed out.

■ MAYO STAND

The mayo stand (Figure 10.17) functions as "instrument central." This is the place where your scrub technician will place the primary instruments that are in use. Instruments come and go from this location and it can be tempting to reach in, take, touch, move, or hand off something. Unless given specific instructions to do so, don't assume that the mayo is a self-service station. All instruments, needles, and sponges have to be accounted for. More hands touching counted items result in a higher likelihood of losing something (or getting stuck by something sharp, which can be very dangerous).

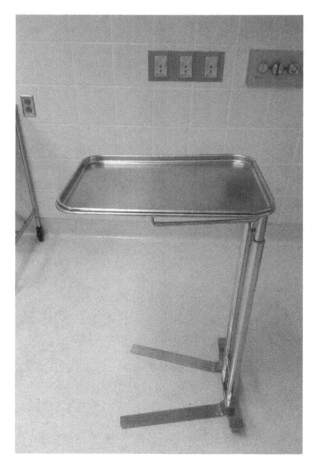

FIGURE 10.17 Mayo stand. (Photo used with permission from Ruth Braga, University of Utah.)

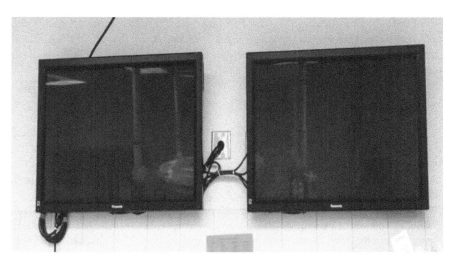

FIGURE 10.18 Monitor screens. (Photo used with permission from Diane Tyler, University of Utah.)

■ MONITORS AND SCREENS

In modern ORs, several screens that look like TV screens hang from the ceiling and can be moved into different positions around the OR table (Figures 10.18 and 10.19). These help the surgeon during laparoscopic or microscopic surgeries. The image from the laparoscopic camera or microscope is displayed on the large-screen TV monitor.

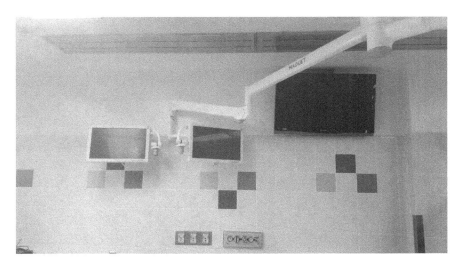

FIGURE 10.19 Monitor and laparoscopy screens. (Photo used with permission from Ruth Braga, University of Utah.)

With the procedure displayed on the overhead screen, the scrub technician can anticipate what instrument the surgeon may need next and the rest of the OR staff can see where the surgeon is in the procedure. These screens are valuable tools for teaching students and other trainees in the operating room.

■ OR BED/REMOTE/CONTROLS

In the center of the room is the OR bed or OR table (Figure 10.20). The surgical patient is brought into the room on a stretcher and is transferred to the table. The table padding is firm and might have a gel pad placed on it for the comfort of the patient (Figure 10.21); it also helps to pad the body to prevent tissue breakdown while the patient is under anesthesia and not moving.

The table can be placed in many positions, depending on the needs of the surgeon and the anesthesiologist. The control (Figure 10.22) will move the table and patient into a position that is best for the intended surgery. The table can be rotated side to side. The patient's head can be moved into a Trendelenburg position (head down) or reverse Trendelenburg position (head up), and the patient's legs can be moved up and down. The table can also be unlocked and moved into a slightly different position within the room depending upon needs for the operation.

■ (BACK) TABLES

There are several instrument tables out of the way of the movement of the OR staff (Figure 10.23). These tables are covered with sterile drapes before the patient is wheeled in, and they hold the sterile instruments and equipment needed for the surgical procedure. The tables remain out of the way until the patient is positioned and surgery is ready to begin. Keeping them out of the way helps decrease the

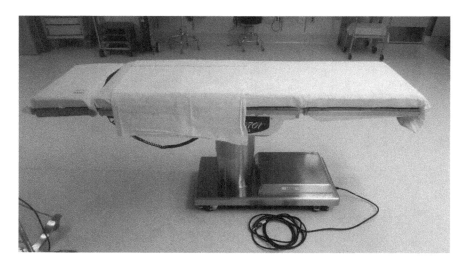

FIGURE 10.20 OR bed without gel pads. (Photo used with permission from Ruth Braga, University of Utah.)

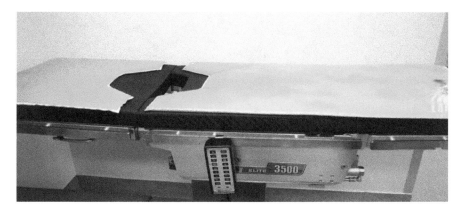

FIGURE 10.21 OR bed with gel pads. (Photo used with permission from Diane Tyler, University of Utah.)

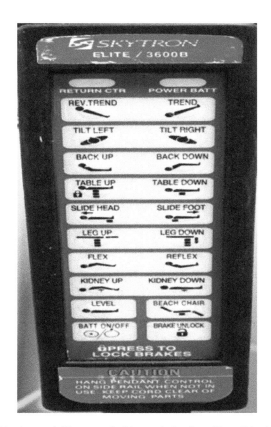

FIGURE 10.22 OR bed control. (Photo used with permission from Diane Tyler, University of Utah.)

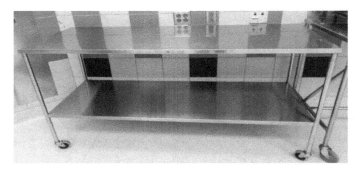

FIGURE 10.23 Long back table for the OR prior to setup. (Photo used with permission from Diane Tyler, University of Utah.)

possibility that one of the OR staff will accidently brush up against the sterile field and contaminate the field.

■ OXYGEN

Similar to air, oxygen is also piped into the operating room. Look for the green lines (Figure 10.24).

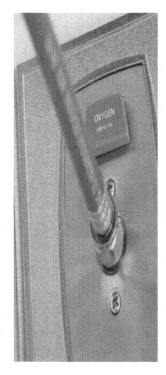

FIGURE 10.24 Oxygen outlet. (Photo used with permission from Diane Tyler, University of Utah.)

■ PREP STAND

The prep stand (Figure 10.25) is a small table that can be used for small setups, such as preparing the patient's skin for surgery. All OR furniture and tables can easily be wiped down before, between, and after cases.

■ RED OUTLETS

These aren't just any electrical outlets. If for some reason the operating room loses power, these are the outlets you need (Figure 10.26). They are powered by the generators and run on backup power. Only the most critical equipment (such as the anesthesia machine) should be plugged into these outlets.

■ RING STANDS

A basic part of standard OR furniture, these stands are just as the name implies: a stand shaped like a ring (Figure 10.27). They provide a steady spot for basins filled with fluid. Some ORs use a variation, such as a double ring stand. These stands are a staple in the OR.

■ ROLLER BOARD

While this is probably one of the most uncomfortable devices ever used to move a patient, the roller board is designed to help save the backs of healthcare workers

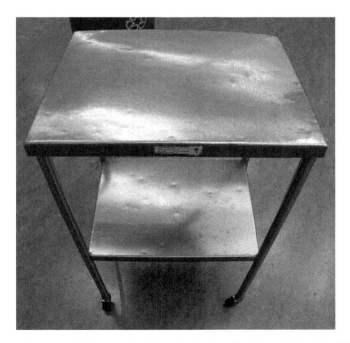

FIGURE 10.25 Prep stand. (Photo used with permission from Ruth Braga, University of Utah.)

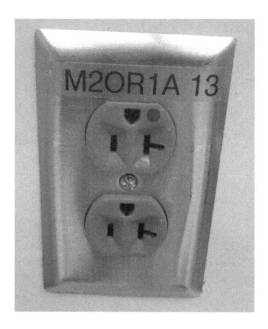

FIGURE 10.26 Red (power failure) outlet. (Photo used with permission from Ruth Braga, University of Utah.)

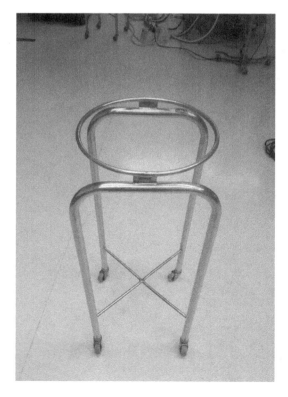

FIGURE 10.27 Ring stand. A bowl of fluids or ice may be seated into this. (Photo used with permission from Ruth Braga, University of Utah.)

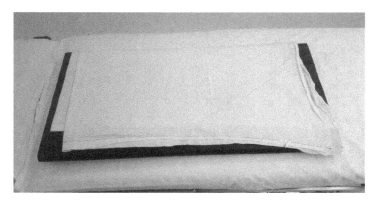

FIGURE 10.28 Roller board set up to move a patient with a sheet. (Photo used with permission from Ruth Braga, University of Utah.)

as we move patients over to the OR bed (Figures 10.28 and 10.29). The sheet is wrapped around one of the long sides of the board and the patient is tipped up on their side and laid back down halfway on the board. As gently as possible, we move the patient from one bed to the other by pulling on that sheet. Use caution and communicate. After you move the patient, this board needs to be pulled out from under the patient. Don't let everyone move on to the next task until this is done.

■ STEP STOOLS

For those who are vertically challenged, or working with those who are vertically gifted, it can be helpful to ask for a step stool (or two) (Figure 10.30). These stackable stools are great if you can't quite reach or see what is going on up at the field. If you are standing on a stool, just remember that you are at a little bit of a higher risk for injury (no pun intended). Don't forget, if you had to step up, you must step down.

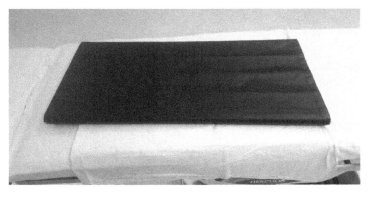

FIGURE 10.29 Roller board without sheet. (Photo used with permission from Ruth Braga, University of Utah.)

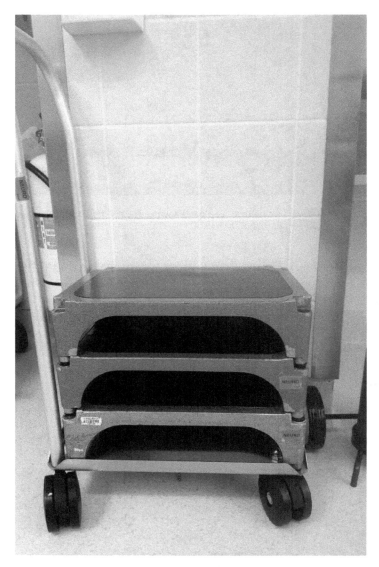

FIGURE 10.30 Step stools (because the entire OR team is not the same height). (Photo used with permission from Ruth Braga, University of Utah.)

■ STRETCHER

Patients roll in, and sometimes out, of the OR on these (Figure 10.31). Since they are notorious for their poor steering, it is always appreciated if you help direct them to where we want them to go. Keep the side rails up during travel and encourage the patient to think of themselves on a ride at the amusement park: hands and legs inside the stretcher at all times. Always remember to lock the wheels on the bed

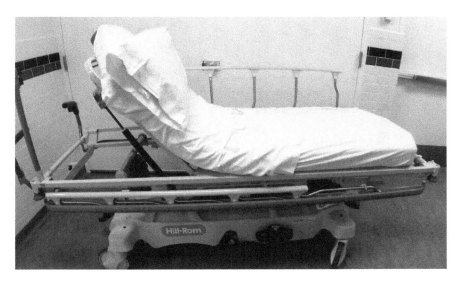

FIGURE 10.31 Stretcher for moving patients to and from the OR. (Photo used with permission from Ruth Braga, University of Utah.)

when you are helping to move the patient. For a bed that is difficult to maneuver, you will be surprised at how well it will maneuver its way straight out from under your patient.

■ SUCTION AND REGULATOR

The suction setup is like an organized octopus (Figure 10.32). This keeps the containers in sight where everyone can see them, and out of the way of accidental kicking. The containers are connected to each other in a way such that when one container is full the fluids flow automatically into the next container. Sometimes it feels as though it is an act of science to get them all properly connected so that the fluid "hops" from canister to canister as intended. If you can't seem to figure out how to set it up, just ask. All fluid is measured and recorded at the end of the procedure. The actual force of suction can be controlled from mild to heavy with the regulator. Tubing goes from the regulator (Figure 10.33) to the canister and then to the surgical field. Avoid tripping on the tubes.

■ SUPPLY CABINETS

No matter how small the OR, it always seems that the central storerooms where disposables, instruments, and surgical packs are kept are massive. To help minimize the need to run in and out of the OR for basic items commonly used, these items are often stocked in the room (Figure 10.34). Before you run out for something, look around and ask because it might already be in the room.

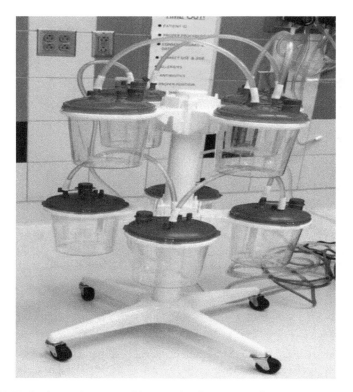

FIGURE 10.32 Suction canister setup. (Photo used with permission from Diane Tyler, University of Utah.)

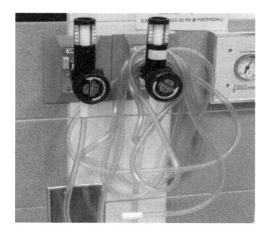

FIGURE 10.33 Suction regulator on the OR wall. (Photo used with permission from Diane Tyler, University of Utah.)

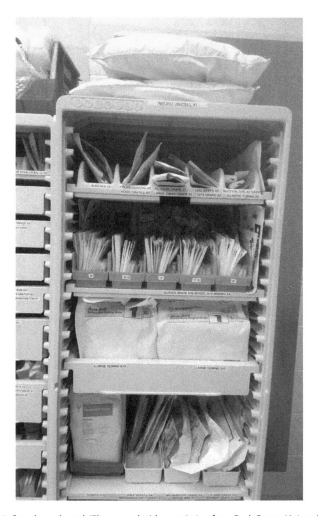

FIGURE 10.34 Supply cupboard. (Photo used with permission from Ruth Braga, University of Utah.)

■ SUTURE (TREE)

Similar to the supply cabinets, some specialties or surgeons use certain suture for many of their cases. Rather than trying to estimate how many packs of such-and-such suture you might need, it is easier to pull the suture tree (Figure 10.35) into— or park it just outside of—the operating room door for access.

■ BLANKET WARMER AND AIR WARMER

The OR is kept on the cool side. This helps the surgical staff stay cool in all of their sterile gowns, but the patient's temperature needs to be maintained. The patient is immobile and does not have the sterile garb of the OR team, and is therefore

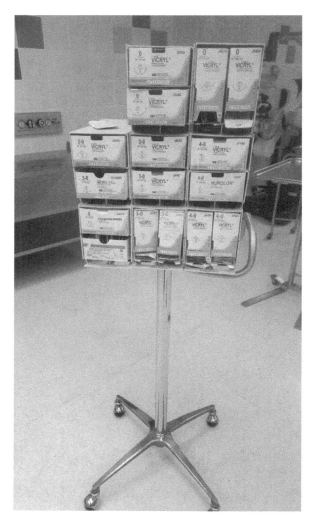

FIGURE 10.35 Suture tree. (Photo used with permission from Ruth Braga, University of Utah.)

unable to maintain a normal body temperature. It is up to the OR staff to ensure the patient stays warm. Cozy, warm blankets and an air warmer (Figures 10.36 and 10.37) are two things that keep the patient warm during surgery. A forced air warmer blows warm air onto the patient through a special blanket with small holes on one side. Warm patients are happy patients.

The operating room is an environment of fascinating things. Keeping them straight may seem like an insurmountable task, but as you gain familiarity with your surroundings and the surgeons you work with, it becomes more manageable.

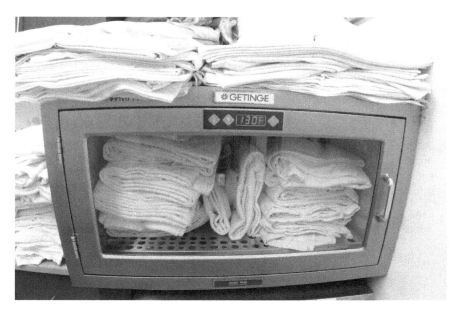

FIGURE 10.36 Blanket warmer (according to patients and Dr. Cochran, the greatest feature of any OR). (Photo used with permission from Ruth Braga, University of Utah.)

Keep learning, take pictures of various setups, and make notes that you can reference when needed. Ask questions. Study the layouts and items used for different procedures. With new procedures, supplies, instruments, and equipment coming out all the time, you will never be bored.

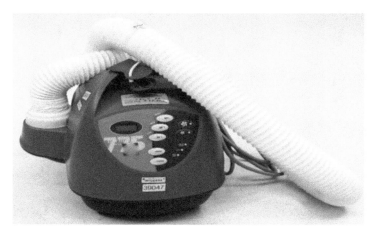

FIGURE 10.37 Forced air warmer. (Photo used with permission from Diane Tyler, University of Utah.)

Robot Basics: The Nurse's Perspective

- *Sebrena Banecker, RN, BSN, CNOR*

I was a semi-experienced new nurse to the OR when first introduced to the robot. It was an intimidating beast weighing over 2000 pounds just for the patient cart. The cords were about an inch around and there were four of them strapped together. The photos that follow were taken by OR staff to demonstrate size, position, and what each component of robot surgery looks like. In an actual case, the cart and patient would be draped, and the scrub technician would be wearing a sterile gown and gloves.

1. **The Patient Cart:** (Figure 10.38) These robotic arms are moved into place to loom over the patient. The arms are draped, and at the direction of the attending

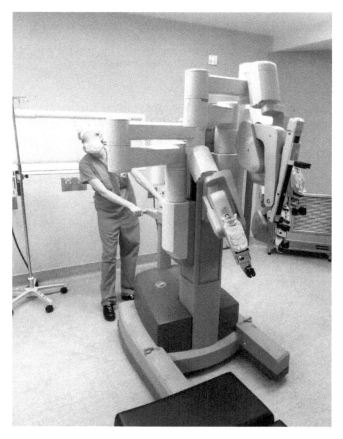

FIGURE 10.38 Positioning the robot and its arms. (Photo used with permission from Walt Medlin, Bariatric Medicine Institute.)

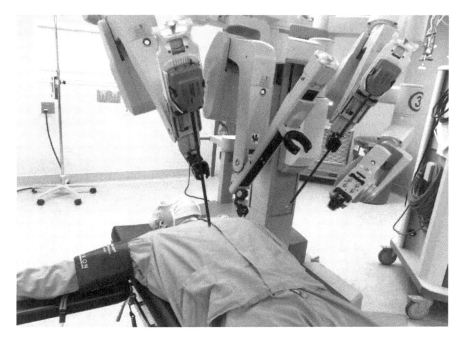

FIGURE 10.39 "Patient" on the OR table positioned for a robotic case. (Photo used with permission from Walt Medlin, Bariatric Medicine Institute.)

surgeon, sterile instruments and devices are placed onto or removed from the arms with the help of the sterile scrub technician or first assist (Figures 10.39 and 10.40).

2. **The Surgeon Console:** The attending surgeon sits here to operate the robotic arms and instruments (Figure 10.41). He/she peers into the console and can see the instruments they are using, the action of their hands, and the patients' anatomy. The surgeon is not scrubbed in or sterile—the case is being controlled by their hands at the console. Every action made by the hand of the surgeon at the console is duplicated by the robotic arm at the patient.

3. **The Video Tower:** This functions as the go-between for the console and patient cart. The scrub technician or first assist and any other staff can watch the tower (Figure 10.42) and anticipate the surgeon's needs or watch as the surgeon explains what he/she is doing.

■ THE SETUP

In earlier models, the cables to set the robot up required a strong back and the ability to solve puzzles: the four-inch plugs had to be plugged into their appropriate colored boxes in just the right order or you would have to start over. After this came the tedious process of draping the patient cart. This required that the drapes be assembled appropriately by the scrub technician, and then placed appropriately.

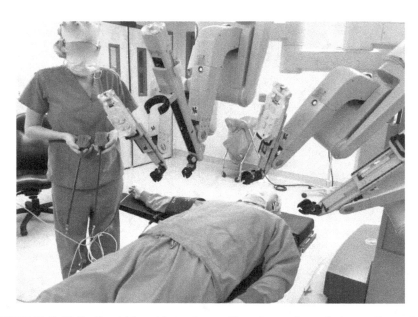

FIGURE 10.40 "Patient" on table and first assistant with equipment for a robotic case. The scrub technician, who will be scrubbed in with the draped sterile robot, will help the surgeon by switching out instruments and assisting as needed. (Photo used with permission from Walt Medlin, Bariatric Medicine Institute.)

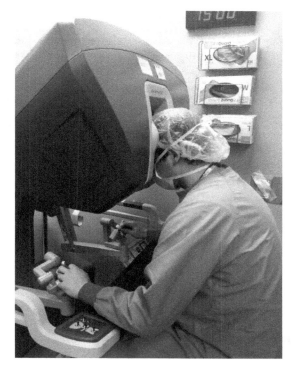

FIGURE 10.41 Surgeon at console. (Photo used with permission from Walt Medlin, Bariatric Medicine Institute.)

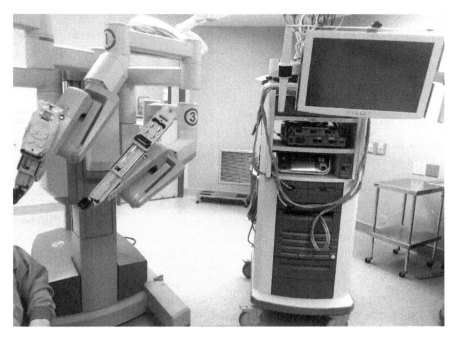

FIGURE 10.42 Tower for a robotic case. This tower will allow the rest of the OR team to see what the surgeon is seeing at the console. (Photo used with permission from Walt Medlin, Bariatric Medicine Institute.)

The camera also had to be draped and assembled. Once this process was completed, the scope had to be calibrated manually at the surgeon console.

Then the "sweet spot": this is the precise position that the robot camera arm must be in for the surgery to be successful. If the camera arm was not precise all bets were off and the surgery was doomed. I still have some anxiety about positioning the arms, but fortunately this does not matter with the new, improved versions. Finally, like steering a boat into the harbor, the robot would be docked. Once docking was successful (sometimes after several attempts), surgery would commence. Many times in the beginning of our robot days, after six or more hours of operating, we would convert to opening the patient and just finish the surgery without the robot.

Improved versions brought sleek, 1-cm single cables in a pretty blue, which could be plugged in to the robot in any order, giving you a rewarding blue wink when you did it correctly. All drapes came assembled with parts that were now disposable (no more signs in the potty reminding all staff which parts of the robot were not disposable). Setup was easy and fast, with amazingly short turnovers, and the dream of three by 3 (three surgery cases by 3:00 p.m.) was born.

■ TODAY

Although it's possible that another version of the robot will come out before this book goes to print, the version we use today is much more user friendly. By moving the pivot point to the top and enabling the entire robot to rotate over the patient, we no longer need to move the bed to crazy places all over the room. The scrub technician is no longer stranded in the corner, and anesthesia is no longer alienated. This has enabled more flexibility in the surgery. By allowing better access to patient anatomy, surgery can be performed more efficiently.

■ APPROACHING THE BEAST

As the new person in the OR, you already have a lot to be aware of. As the new person in the robotic OR, you really need to be alert. Whether you are scrubbed in or observing, being mindful of the robot is the most important thing. Everyone knows that blue or green drapes in the OR means that they are sterile and shouldn't be touched. However, the robot is draped in clear drapes, making it ripe for contamination. When we started working with the robot, contaminating it guaranteed your spot on a "Wanted" poster. Parts had to be re-sterilized, and the case would have to be delayed. These days, you might get a grumble, but re-draping is pretty simple and quick. The only sterile part of the robot is the patient cart with its four arms (Figure 10.43).

If you are in an OR with many residents you will most likely be assigned to a stool. The nice thing about the robot is that optics are great and you will have a bird's-eye view of what is going on. Because the robot has the capability to steady and stabilize the image it is easy to watch and does not induce vertigo like laparoscopic surgery tends to (Figure 10.44).

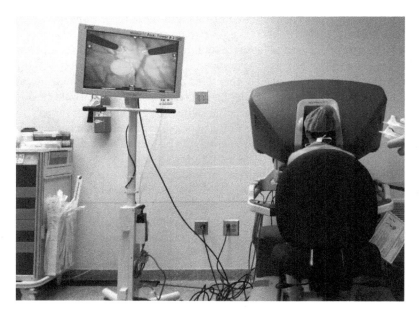

FIGURE 10.43 Robot simulation. (Photo used with permission from Walt Medlin, Bariatric Medicine Institute.)

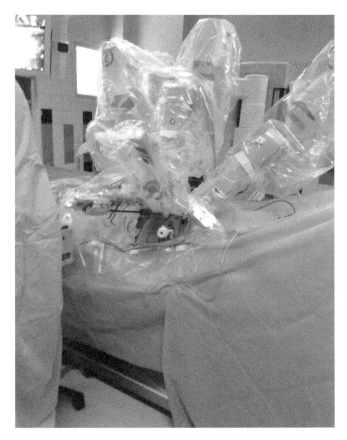

FIGURE 10.44 Case setup with a robot. (Photo used with permission from Daniel Vargo, MD; University of Utah.)

If you are in a not-so crowded OR you might get to scrub in. If you do scrub in, you have to develop great "duck-and-dodge" technique. The arms of the robot can move very swiftly and suddenly and an unsuspecting person will get a smack upside the head. By paying close attention you will see them coming and avoid a concussion. The newer version tends to move in more subtle planes, dramatically decreasing the odds of getting smacked, but you still need to be alert.

When surgery concludes, the arms will be pulled up and away from the patient, instruments disconnected from the cart, and the cart will be moved back, away from the patient. The end of robotic surgery is much like any laparoscopic surgery: trocars are removed, the resident or attending surgeon scrubs in to suture and dress the port sites, and the patient is woken up by anesthesia and rolled out of the OR on a stretcher or hospital bed over to the recovery room.

If you get the opportunity to go to a robotic OR, take advantage of the learning opportunity to witness this amazing technology, watch your head and how you move, and remember, even though robotic surgery may look imposing, you have nothing to fear (from the robot).

My Robot Experience, or How Surgeons Learn New Techniques

* *Walter Medlin, MD, FACS*

My surgical training and career have taken place during the thick of the evolution of minimal invasion. Surgeons in Seattle were adopting laparoscopy for gallbladder disease during my third year med school rotation. I drove the pixelated rod lens laparoscope as experienced open surgeons struggled with early cases using first-generation tools while watching images that varied in quality. They didn't yell much but we all had moments of extreme frustration, and a very real fear that the patient might be at more risk rather than less. There were no simple answers for judgment—and I now understand that is an ongoing challenge for all of us.

Not every advance is an improvement. Hype is rampant, whether for commerce or enthusiasm or professional ambition. Industry commerce is often easy to blame, and practice development pressure can lead to feeling overextended beyond one's ability, and may result in jealousy and criticism as others innovate and try new things. Technology is now significantly more evolved than those early lap cholecystectomies I saw as a medical student, although we are far from done with the evolution of laparoscopic techniques and tools. Flexible endoscopic and transluminal interventions are in their relative infancy, similar to those lap cholecystectomies from my med school days.

Controversy exists on multiple fronts regarding appropriate cost versus value, the degree of risk generated by less invasive techniques, and time required for an evolving technique versus the quicker time of an established technique. Objections to the adoption of new technology are based upon outcomes data ("Is there science to support this decision?"), patient informed consent ("How many of these have you done, doctor?"), staff training ("Hey, who knows how to work this thing?"), and even the "turf" of a particular surgeon ("Should Dr. Q really be doing that procedure?").

My robotic practice grew out of advanced laparoscopic training for bariatric surgery and suturing. I had previously completed robotic coursework in ventral hernia, groin hernia, common bile duct exploration, colon surgery, and anti-reflux surgery.

During a "Top Gun" six-week mini-fellowship in 2003, we had a dry lab day on a first-generation daVinci robot. It rebooted software at least twice every hour we were there—the total blackout of tools and visualization during the reboot could take several minutes, and scared me to death thinking about it happening in the OR. I was glad to know that academic surgeons and engineers were advancing the field, but I was not ready to go further until the tool was more reliable. You never know if that will be weeks, months, or years.

Once I had done 1000 laparoscopic bariatric cases, it seemed like a good time to start looking more seriously at the robot again. During that time, urology had moved to performing greater than 90 percent of prostatectomies robotically in the

United States. Academic centers were starting to develop techniques to use the robot in general surgery, and a few leaders had reported extensive series of patients with excellent outcomes in bariatric surgery. Also, the tool was evolving, and a robotic controllable stapler was on its way (that has since arrived). Is this new, expensive, fancy toy going to help me improve the care of my bariatric surgery patients? Possibly, and I thought it was worth a try.

Still, it took time to get training arranged, and work with our hospital on credentialing, block time, and equipment lists (refined as we trained and networked). Networking is critical for expansion of scope of practice. I consulted with friends and experts at conferences and kept an eye on the literature, in both peer-reviewed and "throwaway" journals. I will admit that the extreme skepticism of questioners at conference presentations and in op-ed pieces was intimidating and made me question whether this was the right practice change. Surgeons are very conservative, and sometimes that valuable caution can become simple obstinacy.

I tried to set my own criteria for use of the robot. What is the goal? Is there a safe pathway? Is there a clearly improved outcome in any subgroup? Can my learning curve occur safely and without absurd cost or effort? Will we ever be able to achieve reasonable speed? The slowest, most risky, most difficult cases for bariatrics are revisions. Previous anti-reflux operations (Nissen fundoplication and hiatal hernia repair) are particularly unforgiving and dangerous. They require open laparotomy far more often, and usually take two to three times longer than "virgin" cases. The robotic tools of 3D visualization, wristed instruments with less torque, and surgeon-controlled camera clearly would give an advantage in my opinion—even if the advantage was limited to less fatigue and better surgeon performance. In my own experience, team performance significantly erodes beyond the 2-hour mark in most cases—and a shaky camera alone can create a spiral of inefficiency, frustration, and compromise.

The steps of adding the skills and experience were challenging, but were almost an afterthought. There are online self-education modules to review, and tests for surgeon safety. I watched as many videos about the optimal positioning of equipment as I did for performing an actual operation. I then took an overnight trip to do case observation with an established robotic general surgeon, followed by full-day lab training at the manufacturer's facility a few weeks later (Figure 10.45).

When I returned from my training, I already had interested patients. I did my first cases with plenty of backup and spare OR time to allow us the freedom to meticulously document and the prep time to confirm our plans. Everyone on the team was involved in room position and case planning—anesthesia, nursing team, scrub techs. We used a combination of expertise from experienced robotic staff with other service lines and our bariatric surgery team. Nothing makes you appreciate the professionalism of a team more than watching them work out a new challenge together. We made sure to have backup equipment to do regular laparoscopy if needed, and had a proctor come twice to observe four cases. He gave us a great custom tutorial for our particular facility and was able to share the perspective from the cutting edge of academia. We started with fairly straightforward cases—trying to learn the machine and the flow of the care—before taking on major challenges.

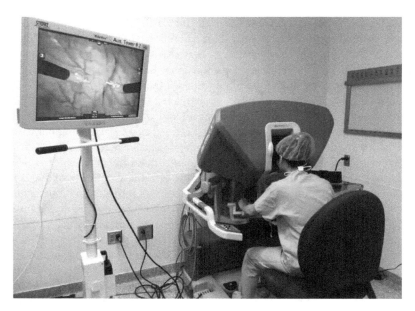

FIGURE 10.45 Using the robot simulator for learning. The picture on the monitor shows what the surgeon is seeing. (Photo used with permission from Walt Medlin, Bariatric Medicine Institute.)

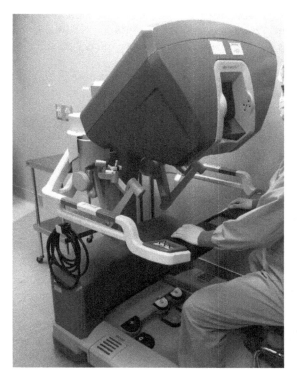

FIGURE 10.46 Surgeon at the robot console and will view the operative site through the lens while maneuvering their hands to operate. (Photo used with permission from Walt Medlin, Bariatric Medicine Institute.)

While it required a generous investment of time for me to launch my robotic career in surgery, the new surgeon who is well supported can get through the training and first five to ten cases in only a few months in the current environment. I have been able to do additional case observation and courses, and have a strong belief that evidence will come for advantage in ventral hernia, groin hernia, and certain colon operations. I have done gallbladder work and trained for single-port technique, but have yet to be convinced to take that step myself. As I had hoped, the robotic staple tool has been more precise than having an assistant firing the handheld device, and as I approach 100 cases over the last 3 years, I truly feel that the advantages are real.

The biggest surprise to me has been patient comfort postoperatively. Supposedly this is due to less torque on the port site at the abdominal wall, a concept I struggle to believe, but patients have clearly been (subjectively) far more comfortable than I expected, even with slightly larger robotic ports compared to standard.

Going forward, I see the robot as a tool to reduce surgeon fatigue, and allow more complex surgery to be done in a given day, and allow surgeons to continue operating for more years as their bodies face the well-documented challenges of repetitive use and ergonomic stress. I also do feel that it reduces patient fear when the surgeon is able to offer more precision and less risk of need to convert to open laparotomy from the standard laparoscopic approach. We still have plenty of learning to do about robotic techniques and their impact, but from my perspective we're off to a great start.

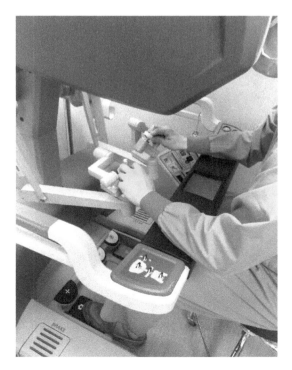

FIGURE 10.47 Surgeon hands on the robot console. Each action of the surgeons' hands are mimicked by the instruments being held by the arms of the robot. (Photo used with permission from Walt Medlin, Bariatric Medicine Institute.)

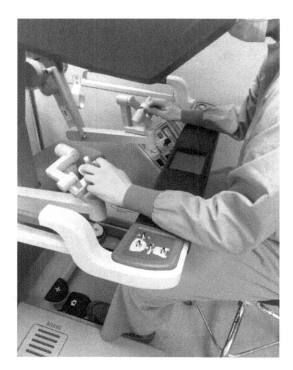

FIGURE 10.48 Foot pedals can be pushed to cauterize tissue as the surgeon gracefully moves their hands to manipulate the surgical instruments. Close-up of surgeon hands on the robot console. (Photo used with permission from Walt Medlin, Bariatric Medicine Institute.)

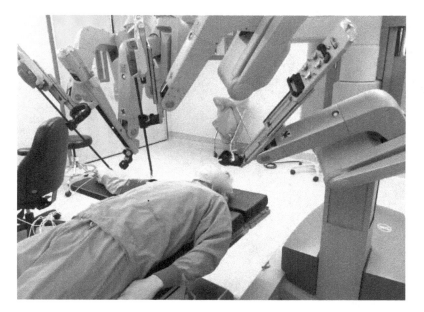

FIGURE 10.49 "Patient" positioned on the table for a robotic case. The robot arms will move the instruments as the surgeons' hands direct them. (Photo used with permission from Walt Medlin, Bariatric Medicine Institute.)

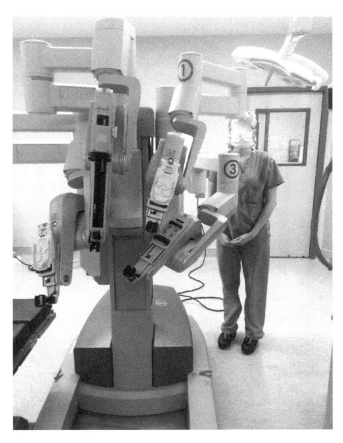

FIGURE 10.50 "Arms" of the robot. (Photo used with permission from Walt Medlin, Bariatric Medicine Institute.)

Dancing Around the Room

- *Ruth Braga, MSN, RN*

Regardless of where you are, there are a few things that are pretty standard on the operating room table. While it is great to be curious, the middle of the case may not be the time to ask what something is or what it does, and you certainly don't want to be caught reaching onto or across the table to answer these questions for yourself (Figure 11.1). Rest assured that no patients, residents, or medical students were harmed in the making of this book. However, if you do not know how to move about the room without touching what shouldn't be touched, I can't make the same promise.

Going to different operating rooms is like visiting different parts of the country. Everyone works for similar outcomes, but the path they take to get there varies by individual. To help you look like a pro, this chapter explains some of the things we do, why we do them, and how you can help us do them. Once again, we want to point out that institutional policies may vary slightly, so always check the policies where you are.

■ THE COUNT

Before you can fully appreciate our obsession over the items found up at the surgical field, you have to know why. Despite modern technology, and as odd as it may seem, leaving behind a sponge or instrument still manages to consistently make it near the top of the list of "Major Mistakes in Medicine" every year. To avoid this, we are number-fixated. There is not a nurse, scrub, resident, or attending who wants to leave something behind in a patient and we will generally do everything possible to keep it from happening. Thus, the count.

Every needle, sponge, instrument, and anything else that could potentially fit into the patient's operative wound must be counted. Not just once, but multiple times. This means before incision and at the end of the case at a minimum. Every

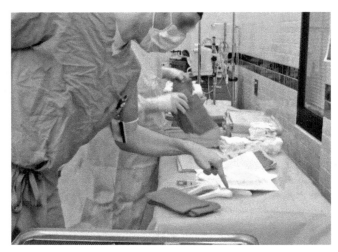

FIGURE 11.1 Don't do this. (Photo used with permission from Ruth Braga, University of Utah.)

number of every item counted at the beginning of the case, plus or minus any items that may have been opened/taken away during the case, must match the numbers at the end of the case. There are no exceptions. If you need something or have a question for your scrub technician or circulator and you hear numbers coming out of their mouths and see papers in hand, do not interrupt. The count requires our full attention.

All instruments that are present prior to a case should be present at the end. As you can see from the list in Figure 11.2, tracking each item (and this is only one pan of instruments) is no small task. Pans come up from the sterile process-ing department with instruments on a "string" consisting of two "rods" that are strung through the handles of each instrument (Figure 11.3). We hope that they are strung in the same order that they are listed on the sheet, as that makes it easier for the scrub technician to quickly move through and announce the amount of each type of instrument, while the circulator follows along in order, with paper and pen in hand. The amount of each type of instrument is noted. The circulator will keep these papers throughout the case and note on the sheet if anything is added or removed.

As the surgeon approaches the closing process, the circulator will pick up that same piece of paper and the scrub technician will organize the instruments once again to prepare for the count. I am always in awe of the scrub technicians at this point. Items have been moved around the field throughout the case and are still in use for the closing process, all while they are counting.

"We're Missing An Instrument"

If the scrub technician states during the closing count that there are four Kelly clamps on the surgical field but the circulator noted there were five at the begin-ning of the case, the OR team is informed that this item is missing and each person

Primary Ster Cycle: **Pre-Vac 270.4.40**   Ster Meth: **Steam**   Manu Proc

Pre Cnt	Cls Cnt	SP Cnt	Qt Mi	Qt Is	Description	Manu	Proc
44					**Stringer: Clamps #1**		
		4		4	Clamp, Mosquito, Curved, 5"	Jarit	107
		4		4	Clamp, Crile, Curved, 5 1/2"	Jarit	107
		4		4	Clamp, Allis, 6"	Jarit	136
		4		4	Clamp, Pean, Curved, 6 1/4"	Jarit	10
		2		2	Clamp, Babcock, 6 1/4"	Jarit	13
		4		4	Clamp, Kocher, Straight, 6 1/4"	Jarit	10
		2		2	Clamp, Pean, Curved, 8"	Jarit	10
		2		2	Clamp, Sarot, Curved, 9 1/2"	Cod	30
		8		8	Clamp, Tonsil, Fully Serrated, Curved, 7 1/2"	AVM	Cl
		4		4	Clamp, Tonsil, Thoracic, Delicate, 9 1/2"	Cod	30
		2		2	Clamp, Allis Willauer, 10"	Jarit	3
		1		1	Clamp, Gemini, Right Angle, 7"	Jarit	1
		2		2	Clamp, Mixter Michigan, Right Angle, 9 1/4"	AVM	
		1		1	Clamp, Kantrowitz, Right Angle, Intestinal, 10 3/4"	Cod	
		2		2	Clamp, Babcock, 9 1/2"	Jarit	
8					**Stringer: Needleholders #2**		
		2		2	Needleholder, Mayo Hegar, 6"	Jarit	
		2		2	Needleholder, Mayo Hegar, 8"	Jarit	
		2		2	Needleholder, Ryder, 2mm, 8"	Jarit	
		2		2	Needleholder, Ryder, 2mm, 10"	Jarit	
6					**Stringer: Scissors #3**		
		1		1	Scissors, Mayo, Curved, 6 3/4"	Jarit	
		1		1	Scissors, Mayo, Straight, 6 3/4"	Jarit	
		1		1	Scissors, Metzenbaum, Curved, 7"	Jarit	
		1		1	Scissors, Metzenbaum, Carbon Edge, Delicate, Curved, 9"	Jarit	
		1		1	Scissors, Metzenbaum, Straight, Delicate, 9"	Jarit	
		1		1	Scissors, Metzenbaum, Curved, 11"	Jarit	
5					**Pan: Towel clamps #4**		
		4		4	Clamp, Towel, Perforating, 5 1/4"	Jarit	
		1		1	Clamp, Towel, Non Perforating, 5 1/4"	Jarit	
2					**Pan: Sponge Sticks**		
		2		2	Clamp, Sponge Stick, Straight, 9"	Jarit	
12					**Pan: Forceps**		
		2		2	Forceps, Adson, w/ Teeth, 5"	Jar	
		2		2	Forceps, Tissue, 6", w/ Teeth	Jar	
		2		2	Forceps, Ferris Smith, 6 3/4"	Jar	
		2		2	Forceps, DeBakey, Regular, 7 3/4"	Ja	
		2		2	Forceps, DeBakey, Heavy, 9 1/2"	Ja	
		2		2	Forceps, DeBakey, Regular, 12"	Ja	
4					**Pan: Knife Handles**		
		2		2	Handle, Knife, #3	Ja	
		1		1	Handle, Knife, #7	Ja	
		1		1	Handle, Knife, #3 Long	Ja	
1					**Pan: Ruler**		
		1		1	Ruler, Metal, 6"	J	

FIGURE 11.2 Instrument list of items in a pan. (Photo used with permission from Ruth Braga, University of Utah.)

will look around them. If you are at the field, carefully look around yourself and lift your feet to see if something fell on the floor. Sometimes an instrument has fallen on the floor without being noticed. If you are scrubbed in and up at the field when an instrument or something else falls, tell the circulator or scrub technician right away that it fell. You will save everyone the search time. If you are not scrubbed in and notice that something has fallen, speak up so it can be set aside and accounted for. Whatever you do, don't throw it out—surgical instruments are very expensive.

Many circulators like to make a special place to put instruments or other items that fell or are no longer in use but still need to be accounted for. Whatever method

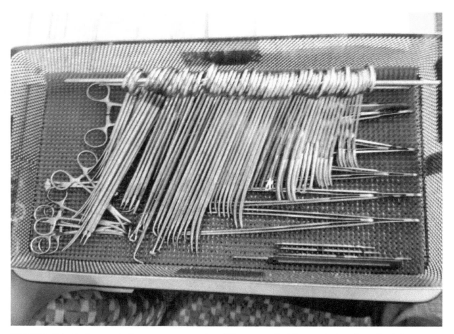

FIGURE 11.3 Instruments for a case on a string. (Photo used with permission from Ruth Braga, University of Utah.)

you use, make sure others know about it. I have crawled around on my hands and knees, dug through trash, and called other nurses or scrub technicians at home to find out where they put something. I've even gone so far as to poke surgeons in the legs to get them to move their feet so I could look for something.

If the missing item is not on the floor, hidden under a drape, or anywhere else to be found, the patient will need an x-ray to make sure the unaccounted-for instrument was not left inside the patient. Institutional policies may vary but in most places if a patient requires an x-ray because an item is missing, they must stay under anesthesia until the x-ray has been taken and read by a radiologist to confirm that the item was not left behind. Incident reports or other reporting may be required, as this can be a serious patient safety issue.

■ SPONGES

Lap sponges are used in many cases. Extremely absorbent, they can be used for just about everything up at the surgical field. In sterile packaging, laps come in packs of five and measure about 10″ × 10″ (Figure 11.4).

Before working in the OR, I always wondered how it was possible for a surgeon to leave a sponge in a patient. Because lap sponges are so absorbent, they can become very bloody, small, and difficult to see. Once they are wadded up, they blend in very well. A nursing student asked me once what the little blue string on the lap sponge was for (Figure 11.5). This strategically placed blue string helps us

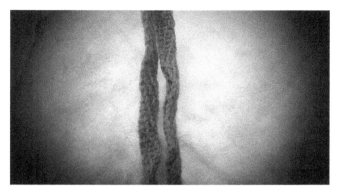

FIGURE 11.4 Laparotomy sponges. (Photo used with permission from Ruth Braga, University of Utah.)

to avoid leaving them behind by making it possible for the sponge to show up on an x-ray. They are also nice to hold on to when a circulator has many to count. Large cases could use well into the hundreds of lap sponges and each individual sponge must be counted; the use of sponge counter bags is helpful because they allow each sponge to be separated out into its own pocket, making it easy for the scrub tech to also see how many sponges the nurse has (Figure 11.6).

A well-intended medical student once caused memorable grief for me as a circulator. Wanting to follow the advice of his preceptors and be helpful, he decided to "clean up." After seeing the resident toss what he thought were sponges into a garbage can, he assumed that all sponges should be tossed. The operative staff does toss the sponges: into the kickbucket (Figure 11.7) for the circulator to pick

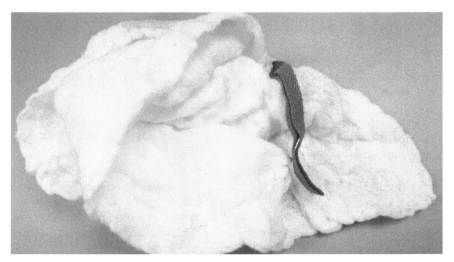

FIGURE 11.5 Close-up view of a laparotomy sponge. (Photo used with permission from Ruth Braga, University of Utah.)

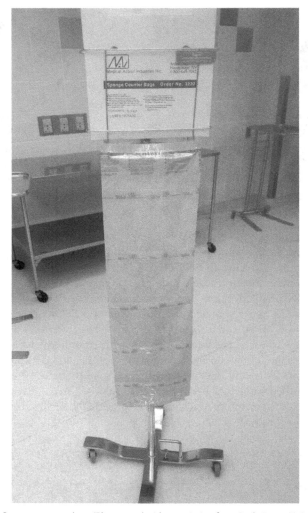

FIGURE 11.6 Sponge counter bag. (Photo used with permission from Ruth Braga, University of Utah.)

up, hang in the sponge counter bag, and count. What this helpful medical student failed to realize is that the sponges he threw out were considered counted sponges and that his actions resulted in a scavenger hunt for the team.

How do you tell the difference as a newbie? Most have variations in packaging, but the key is that counted sponges have that blue squiggly line that runs through the weave (Figures 11.8 and 11.9). This blue line serves the same purpose as the blue string in the lap sponge: they will show up on x-ray if accidentally left behind. These are the only sponges that should be open anywhere in the room once an incision has been made. Each one has to be accounted for, and there will be some serious dumpster diving taking place if the final sponge count doesn't match what is recorded on paper.

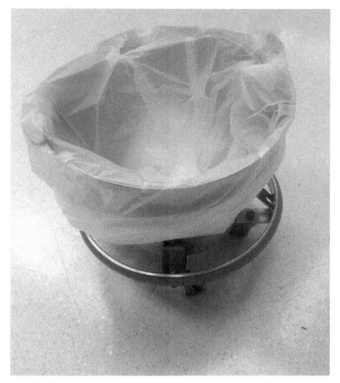

FIGURE 11.7 Kickbucket. (Photo used with permission from Ruth Braga, University of Utah.)

Sometimes the sponges pictured here (Figure 11.10) are used to prep or for dressing and can be confused with counted sponges, and vice-versa. These sponges should not be on the field with an open incision. I personally don't even like them open in the room.

■ SHARPS

Needles and the suture attached to them come in a variety of sizes. However, all needles have one thing in common: they are small enough to be left behind in a person. To prevent this and make it possible to account for each of the sometimes hundreds that are opened, the scrub technician will use a sharps container to store them during the case (Figure 11.11). This numbered pincushion provides a quick, at-a-glance view at how many needles have been used. How they are sorted is up to the tech or institutional policy. If you are opening a packet of suture to be placed on the operative field, remember that suture comes in single or multi-packs. Double-check the packaging so you know how many needles you or the circulator need to track. When these are dropped or lost, they can be very difficult to find, and depending on size, particularly small ones may not show up on x-ray.

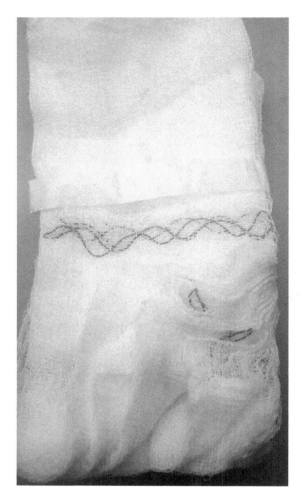

FIGURE 11.8 Package of Raytech sponges. (Photo used with permission from Ruth Braga, University of Utah.)

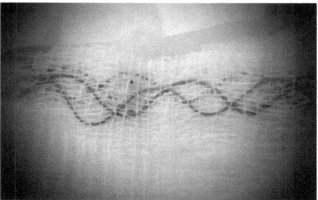

FIGURE 11.9 Close-up view of a Raytech sponge. (Photo used with permission from Ruth Braga, University of Utah.)

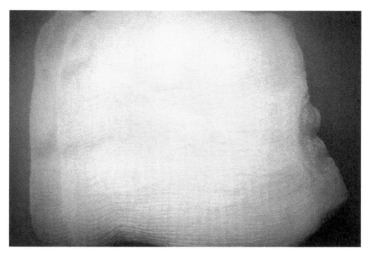

FIGURE 11.10 Gauze dressing. (Photo used with permission from Ruth Braga, University of Utah.)

Some ORs have a magnet on wheels that the circulator will push (similar to a push broom), "sweeping" around the floor of the OR bed and instrument table to pick them up. Just watch your ankles if the circulator gets this device out—it really hurts to be slammed into by one of these.

■ INSTRUMENTS

As noted, all instruments must be accounted for. At first glance, you may wonder how to tell the difference between them, since so many of the instruments look the same. Handles may look the same (Figure 11.12), but it is the tip of the instrument that

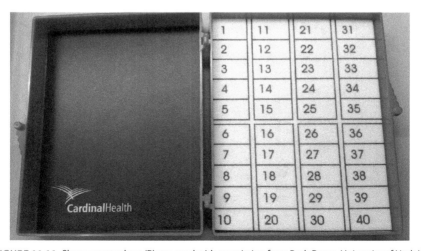

FIGURE 11.11 Sharp counter box. (Photo used with permission from Ruth Braga, University of Utah.)

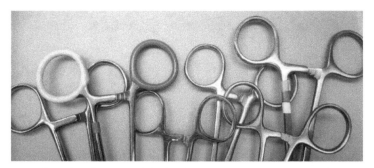

FIGURE 11.12 Clamp handles—they all look alike. (Photo used with permission from Ruth Braga, University of Utah.)

makes the difference (Figure 11.13). Learning the names and functions can be difficult and will take time (and is beyond the scope of your introduction to the OR).

■ FLUIDS AND MEDICATIONS

Normal saline and water are probably the two most commonly used fluids on the scrub technician's table. There is definitely a potential problem here: there is no visual difference between the two. Since we don't want to use water when we should be using saline, and vice-versa, there are usually sterile stickers or labels available in basic packs (Figure 11.14). The scrub technician will use these to label the basins so they know which is which. In longer cases, a fluid warmer may be used instead of a basin on the back table (see Chapter XX). Be mindful of what you touch—this warmer will be draped in a clear plastic drape, but it is still sterile.

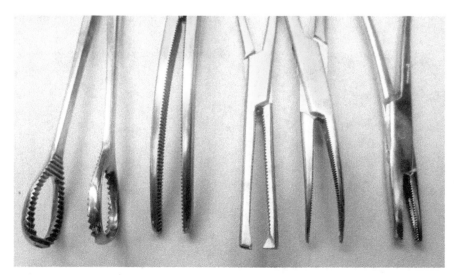

FIGURE 11.13 Clamp tips—they don't look so much alike. (Photo used with permission from Ruth Braga, University of Utah.)

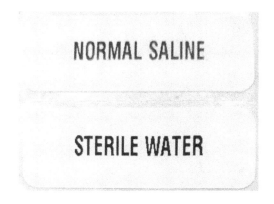

FIGURE 11.14 Labels for fluid basins. (Photo used with permission from Ruth Braga, University of Utah.)

Medications must also be clearly labeled. Often, the circulator draws up the medication from the original packaging using a needle and syringe, and then shoots it into a sterile cup on the scrubs table. Because it is out of its packaging, it needs to be clearly labeled so that anyone who came in to that OR would be able to see what is on the table. Pay attention to the labels and keep your patient safe.

■ STAPLE IT UP

Skin staplers are considered one of the most useful tools on the OR table (Figure 11.15). These disposable staplers can be used for stapling drapes around (or onto) the patient or fixing a towel into place. With a pair of forceps in one hand and a stapler in the other, it is used to close the skin. If the incision is large, you may need a few of them. Often residents will allow medical students to assist with this part of the case. If you look for the tiny line at the tip of the stapler and center it with the incision, your placement of the staples will be a bit more aesthetically pleasing.

This overview shows only a small portion of the items you may find in the OR. Keep asking questions (appropriately timed), and speak up if you notice something that other staff members didn't. We will appreciate your help, and it tells us you are paying attention to what's happening around you.

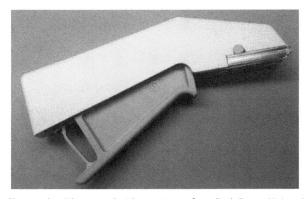

FIGURE 11.15 Skin stapler. (Photo used with permission from Ruth Braga, University of Utah.)

CHAPTER 12

The OR and The Surgical Field

• *Karen Porter, BSN, RN*

The surgical field is the sterile field that is set up by the scrub tech and consists of the draped patient, the back table, and any equipment that is draped out, such as microscopes, slush machines, and c-arms. The scrub tech will open the field, supplies, and instruments and then scrub in. Once they are scrubbed they will self-gown and glove and begin the setup process (Figure 12.1). The goal is to create and maintain a sterile environment for the patient.

Whether you are scrubbing in or coming to observe for a case in the operating room, there are a few things that everyone has to do before "crossing over" into the actual operating rooms:

1. In the operating room dressing area, change into hospital-issued OR scrubs. No shirt should be worn under the scrub top—nothing should be hanging out from the sleeves or neck.
2. Remove jewelry and put it somewhere secure so you don't lose it. Allowing earrings and necklaces in the OR is a hot topic of debate, so always check with your facility. If earrings are allowed, be sure they are secure and are covered by your hat. No one wants to search through an open abdomen for your earring because the back fell off (yes, it has happened).
3. Dedicated OR footwear or shoe covers should be worn. You don't want to bring anything from home into the OR and you certainly don't want to take anything from the OR into your home.
4. Put on a clean hat. The hat must cover all hair and for that reason many facilities no longer allow skullcaps. And don't forget a mask.
5. Do not bring bags or other personal belongings into the operating room. It is a clean environment, and bags and other items bring microorganisms in.
6. When you enter the OR, introduce yourself to the circulating nurse (at a minimum). If you haven't met the surgeon before, it's your responsibility to introduce yourself and tell them why you are there.

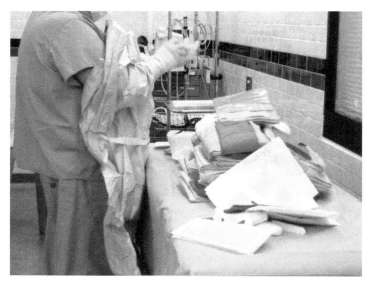

FIGURE 12.1 Scrub tech placing his own gown and gloves on to prepare for a case. (Photo used with permission from Ruth Braga, University of Utah.)

■ IF YOU ARE OBSERVING

If you are not going to be putting a gown and gloves on but are coming to watch the case, there are some important tips to remember:

1. Non-scrubbed staff should stay at least 12 inches away from the sterile field at all times. If it's blue and you're not scrubbed, it's not for you.
2. Never cross between two sterile fields. For example, if you need to go to the other side of the room, don't cut between the instrument table and the draped OR bed. Always go completely around.
3. Do not turn your back to the sterile field. Always be mindful of where you are in relation to it.
4. Excess traffic should be minimized, including people coming and going from the OR. This increases the risk of contamination and is a source of distraction to the surgical team. If you have to go to a different OR for some reason, use the side doors when possible.
5. Keep conversations to a minimum. If everyone around the patient is quiet and focusing only on the case, it's probably not the best time to ask questions.

All of this is really challenging. You will ask (and be asked) a lot of questions. Just do your best.

■ IF YOU ARE SCRUBBING IN

Before you scrub, double check that the following things are done:

1. Your mask is on properly, covering both the nose and mouth, and tied tightly. Beard covers should be worn as needed.

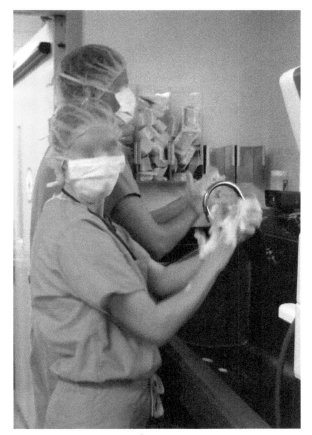

FIGURE 12.2 Medical students scrubbing in. Don't forget to put your goggles on your face before you scrub! (Photo used with permission from Ruth Braga, University of Utah.)

2. Protective eye gear is on, not resting on your forehead or waiting on the counter for you to put it on (Figure 12.2).
3. If you are going into an OR where x-ray will be used, select a lead apron and put that on before you scrub.
4. Remove all cell phones and pagers from your pockets. The circulator really doesn't enjoy having to reach under your gown to find your phone when it rings during the case and you forgot to put it on the counter.

■ HOW TO SCRUB IN

Always follow specific hospital policies on how to scrub in.

1. A surgical scrub is performed on clean hands. If hands are soiled they must be pre-washed.
2. Fingernails should be short and clean. No nail polish or artificial nails are allowed at many facilities. If you have cuts or abrasions on your hands or arms, you should not scrub in.

3. Clean fingernails of both hands under running water with a disposable nail cleaner.
4. Rinse hands and arms with running water.
5. Dispense antimicrobial cleaning agent.
6. Apply antimicrobial agent to wet hands and forearms using a soft sponge. You will need plenty of soapy water to work with: place the sponge under water and squeeze it to get more soap as needed.
7. A three- to five-minute scrub is performed according to manufacturer's guidelines (Figure 12.3).
8. Each finger, hand and arm has four sides. Scrub all four sides, keeping hands elevated at all times (Figure 12.4).
9. Repeat for the opposite side. Wash arms to 2 inches above the elbow.
10. Please turn water off when you aren't using it to help conserve this resource.
11. Avoid splashing your attire.
12. Discard the scrub sponge in the trash.

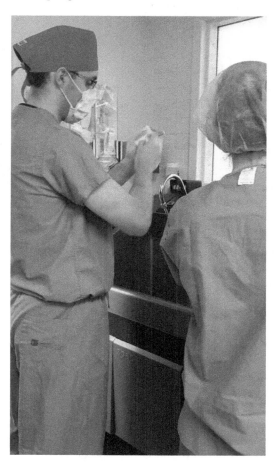

FIGURE 12.3 A good scrub is a critical step to keeping your patient infection-free. (Photo used with permission from Ruth Braga, University of Utah.)

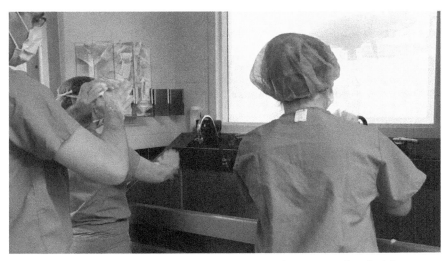

FIGURE 12.4 Hands stay elevated at all times. (Photo used with permission from Ruth Braga, University of Utah.)

13. Rinse hands and arms under running water in one direction, from fingertips to elbows.
14. Keep hands and fingertips higher than your elbows and away from attire at all times.

In many facilities, it is also acceptable to use a "waterless scrub" (Figure 12.5). Check your facility policy to determine if it can be used as the first scrub of the day. Directions for using a waterless scrub are as follows:

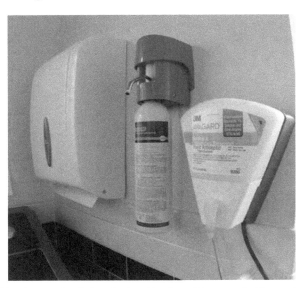

FIGURE 12.5 Waterless scrub solutions for hand hygiene. (Photo used with permission from Ruth Braga, University of Utah.)

1. Use on clean, dry hands.
2. Dispense one pump of the solution into hand, dip fingertips of the opposite hand into the solution and work under fingernails. Spread the remaining solution over your hand and up to 2 inches above the elbow.
3. Dispense one pump of the solution into opposite hand and repeat.
4. Dispense an additional pump into either hand. Rub it into hands up to wrists until it is dry.
5. Do not use towels. You will proceed into the OR, following the steps below, with the exception of Step 4 below.

Scrubbing takes longer than you think when you first start. Practice is the key. We have all been there and made mistakes. Ask for help—it is ok.

■ WHEN YOU HAVE COMPLETED THE SCRUB

1. Walk into the OR using your backside to open the door, keeping your hands up and in front of you (Figures 12.6 and 12.7).
2. Carefully enter without bumping into objects or equipment inside the OR.

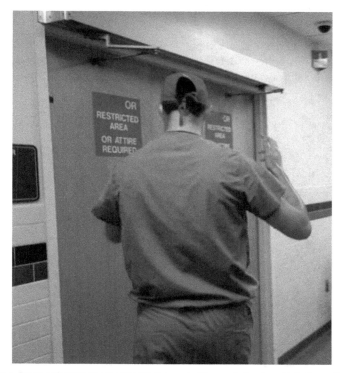

FIGURE 12.6 Post-scrub: entering the OR. (Photo used with permission from Ruth Braga, University of Utah.)

3. Once you are in the OR, go straight to the back table to get a towel from the scrub technician to dry your hands and arms thoroughly (unless waterless scrub has been used; see above). If the scrub technician is busy, you may need to wait or do this yourself, but always ask before reaching and taking a towel or gown from the sterile field. If you are responsible for getting your own towel, remember to go to the edge of the back table to get it—don't drip on the sterile instruments.

4. When drying your hands, use a different part of the towel for each hand (Figures 12.8 through 12.12). Do you notice a potential problem in Figure 12.12? The student has not removed her pager—hopefully it won't go off from under her gown.

5. The scrub technician will hold the gown for you, with the interior of the gown facing you. Keeping your hands up and out, extend arms into the armholes of the gown and simultaneously push your hands into the sleeves and out away from the scrub technician (Figure 12.13).

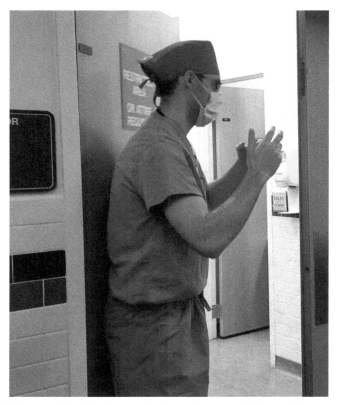

FIGURE 12.7 Post-scrub, backing through the doors. (Photo used with permission from Ruth Braga, University of Utah.)

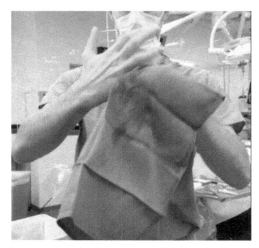

FIGURE 12.8 Drying hands post-scrub. (Photo used with permission from Ruth Braga, University of Utah.)

6. Do not allow your fingertips to extend past the cuff of the gown. When you feel the material of the cuff, it's time to stop pushing your hands through. (Figure 12.14)
7. The circulator or other non-sterile person will come behind you and tie up the back of your gown (Figure 12.15)

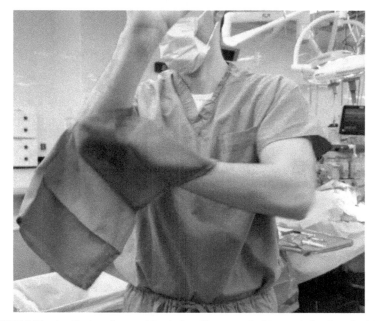

FIGURE 12.9 Turning the towel around for drying. (Photo used with permission from Ruth Braga, University of Utah.)

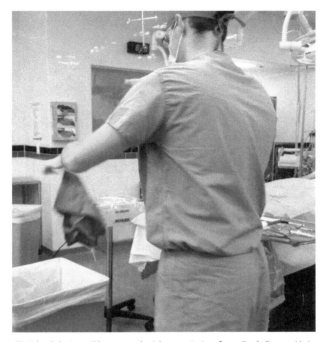

FIGURE 12.10 Finished drying. (Photo used with permission from Ruth Braga, University of Utah.)

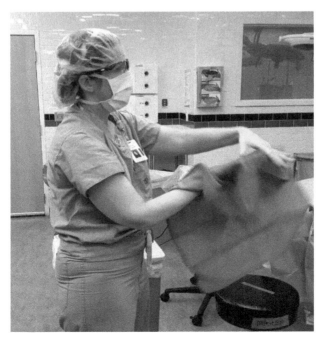

FIGURE 12.11 Attending drying hands for the case. (Photo used with permission from Ruth Braga, University of Utah.)

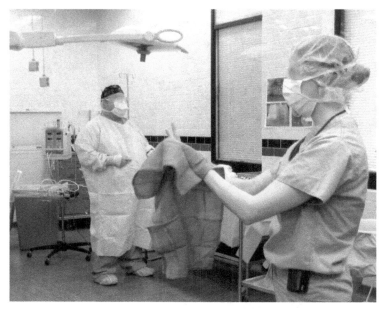

FIGURE 12.12 Don't forget to remove your pager! (Photo used with permission from Ruth Braga, University of Utah.)

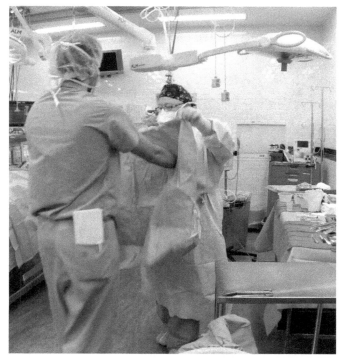

FIGURE 12.13 Gowning for the case. (Photo used with permission from Ruth Braga, University of Utah)

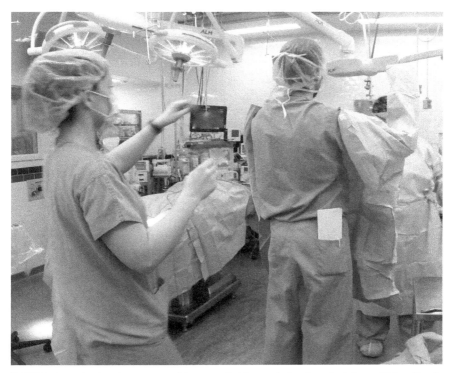

FIGURE 12.14 Getting the gown on. (Photo used with permission from Ruth Braga, University of Utah.)

8. The scrub technician will hold out the right-hand glove for you. Bring your fingertips to the very edge of the cuff of the gown, and "dive" into the glove, pushing your fingertips out of the gown and into the glove at the same time.
9. The scrub technician will hold out the left glove for you. With your right hand, reach under the folded cuff of the left glove, and pull it toward you. Bring the fingertips of the left hand to the edge of the gown cuff, and "dive" your left hand into the glove.
10. Your gloves are now on and you can adjust them as necessary. The cuff of your gown should be completely covered by the glove and not exposed. It is up to you and your facility, but we recommend that you double glove for your safety (Figures 12.16 and 12.17).
11. The scrub technician, circulator, resident (anyone in the OR) will then ask you to "dance," "spin," or "turn" (Figure 12.18). No, this is not a proposition. They are asking you to take the card and tie that is on the front of the gown, hand it off to them, and turn so the tie goes around you and closes the gown behind you. Once this is complete, you are ready to approach the sterile field.

If you are unsure about where to stand at the OR table (or within the OR if you aren't scrubbed), just ask. Scrubbed team members should remain close to sterile

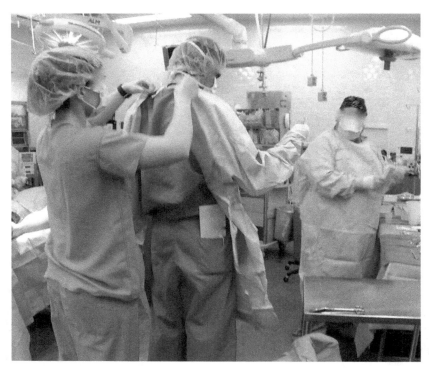

FIGURE 12.15 Tying up the gown. (Photo used with permission from Ruth Braga, University of Utah.)

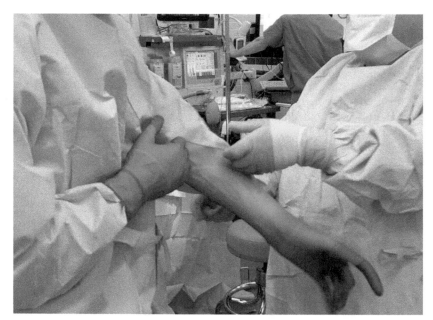

FIGURE 12.16 Gloving with "indicator" gloves. (Photo used with permission from Ruth Braga, University of Utah.)

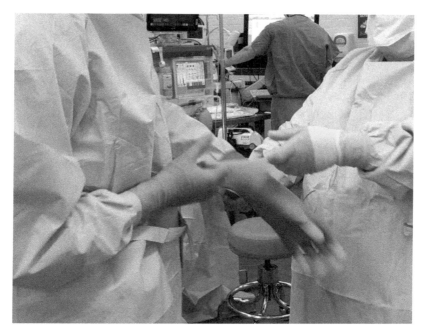

FIGURE 12.17 Double-gloving for safety. (Photo used with permission from Ruth Braga, University of Utah.)

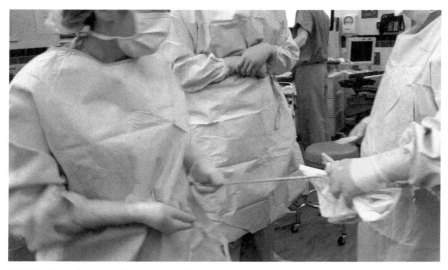

FIGURE 12.18 "Spinning" in the gown. (Photo used with permission from Ruth Braga, University of Utah.)

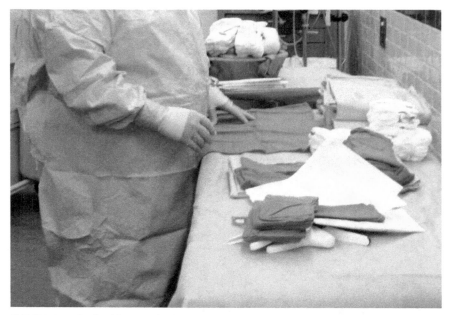

FIGURE 12.19 Back-table set up by the scrub technician. (Photo used with permission from Ruth Braga, University of Utah.)

field (Figure 12.19) and should minimize movement about the room. Keep your hands above the level of your waist and below the nipple line. If they leave that zone, they are no longer considered sterile. Don't put your gloved hands into your armpits, and don't dangle them.

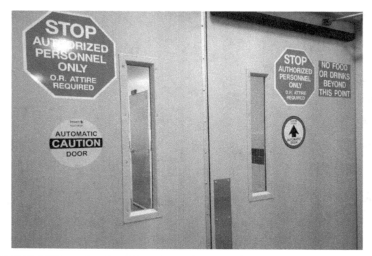

FIGURE 12.20 OR Doors: in spite of those signs, it's amazing how many people will try to get in here! (Photo used with permission from Ruth Braga, University of Utah.)

If you are asked to trade places with the surgeon or someone else at the field, use caution and carefully walk around the sterile field, facing it at all times. When you pass someone, go face-to-face or back-to-back, and always be aware of your surroundings.

If you contaminate something or notice that something has been contaminated, speak up. We can fix it. But we need to know. We don't want our patient to get an infection. What about if the attending surgeon contaminates something? Discreetly mention it to the scrub tech or the circulator. We will take care of it. Just tell us. Medical, nursing, and scrub tech students often notice things that might have been overlooked or unnoticed. Tell us. We are advocates for the patient's safety, which is the commitment of the entire team. If you don't feel comfortable addressing an issue we will.

And one very important item: If you start to feel at all lightheaded during a case, back away from the field and say something to the circulator. You need to get into a seated position and/or outside of the room ASAP. It's better to have a "near miss" than to fall out during the case.

Remember, this entire process can take multiple attempts to master. Don't give up, ask questions, and be sure to communicate with the staff in your operating room.

Although the OR can be intimidating from the first point of entry, we need you to help the team. Speak up if you have questions or notice that something isn't right-everyone will appreciate it! (Figure 12.20).

CHAPTER 13

Lines and Tubes: What Are All of Those Things Sticking Out of the Patient's Body?

- *Halle Kogan BSN, RN, CCRN and Thaona D. Garber, RN*

Lines and tubes come in a variety of shapes and sizes, and for varied purposes. You may see any (or all) of these lines and tubes in the OR, and may even be asked to get one or help put one into the patient. Let's cover some important basic things you need to know.

■ PERIPHERAL IVS

Peripheral IVs (Figure 13.1) come in various sizes, referred to as gauges. Don't ask us why, but the bigger the IV, the smaller the number. A good size for an IV in an adult is at least an 18 or 20 gauge, because red blood cells fit through that size. You can place an IV in any vein, but typical sites are the hands and forearms. A lot of IVs that get placed in the emergency department go into the antecubital vein, which ICU nurses hate because the patient inevitably bends his or her arm, causing the IV pump to go off repeatedly. Peripheral IVs should be placed using aseptic technique, and most hospitals have an IV care protocol for nursing. Fluid, blood, and blood products and many medications can be administered intravenously through a peripheral IV. There are many drugs that cannot be given through a peripheral IV, including chemotherapy drugs and very strong antibiotics that can damage the vein. For these IV medications, central venous access is preferred.

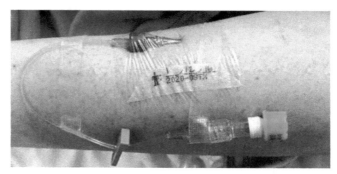

FIGURE 13.1 Peripheral IV. (Photo used with permission from Amalia Cochran, MD, University of Utah.)

■ INTRAOSSEOUS CATHETER

An intraosseous catheter (IO) is a great way to gain access for fluids and medications very quickly. This is a good tool if your patient is a difficult stick with a regular peripheral IV. The IO might be an option in the obese patient, pediatric patient, the elderly patient (who may have tortuous veins that roll), and the burn patient. An IO is drilled directly into the bone using a device that looks like a hot glue gun. While this sounds pretty awful, patients say it's not as painful as you would expect. A common place to put in an IO is the tibial plateau. Placing one of these gives you 24 hours to place a peripheral or central line and is a great tool in an emergency setting.

■ MIDLINE CATHETER

A midline catheter is an 8- to 20-cm small diameter tube that is inserted into a vein in the upper arm and terminates in the axillary vein. It is inserted with ultrasound guidance under sterile conditions. It is used to deliver fluids, antibiotics, and other medications to patients. This device does not provide central access but it can be left in for an indefinite time period, in contrast to a regular peripheral IV that needs to be changed every few days.

■ ARTERIAL LINE

Arterial lines (Figure 13.2) provide a continuous blood pressure reading and allow for blood to be drawn directly from an artery. Arterial lines are particularly useful in a critically ill patient where organ perfusion is a concern and accurate measurement of blood pressure is essential for titration of pressors. They are typically inserted into a radial or femoral artery and hooked to a pressure bag and a transducer that transmits information to a monitor to get a waveform reading of systolic, diastolic, and mean arterial pressures. Also, it is extremely easy to draw blood gases and other labs from an arterial line without the patient needing to be stuck with a needle. Blood gases can be drawn frequently on ventilated patients

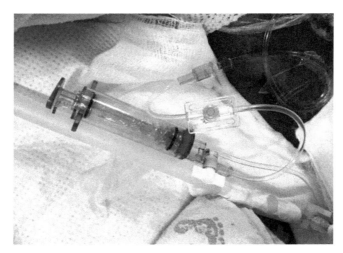

FIGURE 13.2 Arterial line and stopcock. (Photo used with permission from Amalia Cochran, MD, University of Utah.)

with minimal blood waste and no additional pain to the patient, which allows us to monitor oxygenation and ventilation in patients with respiratory failure.

■ CENTRAL VENOUS CATHETER

A central venous catheter (CVC), or central line (Figure 13.3), is a small diameter tube placed into the venous system and terminates in a central vessel that delivers blood directly to the heart, either the superior or inferior vena cava. The three usual sites of insertion are the jugular, subclavian, or femoral vein. The size of the vessel and volume of blood at the terminal site allows a CVC to safely carry chemotherapy medications or fluids of extreme pH that can be harmful to the smaller peripheral vessels. The body then distributes the fluid systemically through the circulatory system. CVCs can have single or multiple lumens (up to five) for noncompatible infusions and drawing blood for laboratory sample.

■ PERIPHERALLY INSERTED CENTRAL CATHETER

The peripherally inserted central catheter (PICC line) (Figure 13.4) is a special type of central venous catheter that is inserted into the basilic or brachial vein and terminates in the superior vena cava. PICC lines may have a single, double, or triple lumen. Each lumen can be utilized for noncompatible medications or drawing blood for laboratory samples. PICC lines provide central venous access in patients who require it without the risks associated with placing a central line.

■ PRESSURE TRANSDUCER

It is not uncommon to see an arterial line, CVC, or PICC connected to a pressure transducer. The transducer is used to determine the blood pressure or the central

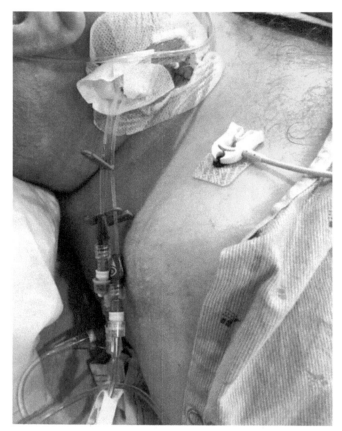

FIGURE 13.3 Right internal jugular central venous catheter and dressing. (Photo used with permission from Amalia Cochran, MD, University of Utah.)

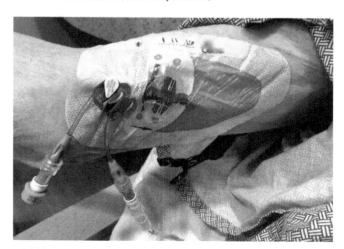

FIGURE 13.4 PICC line and dressing. (Photo used with permission from Amalia Cochran, MD, University of Utah.)

venous pressure (CVP). For CVP, a higher pressure indicates a large volume of fluid returning to the heart, or the preload. This number is trended over time and helps the medical team to determine the fluid status of a patient. A low trending number can indicate the need to administer more IV fluid. A high trending number can indicate the need to reduce the amount of fluid in the patient's venous system, usually by reducing the amount of fluid being administered, and sometimes by giving diuretics. A normal range of CVP for a healthy individual is 6–8 mmHg.

■ SWAN-GANZ CATHETER

A Swan-Ganz catheter (also called a pulmonary artery catheter [PAC]) is a thin plastic tube that is placed into the patient's venous system, usually through an "introducer" to the central venous system, and travels through the heart and to the arteries leading to the lungs. This catheter enters the right atrium, travels past the tricuspid valve into the right ventricle, past the pulmonic valve into the pulmonary artery. It is connected to a transducer that can determine the volume of fluid and pressure within the heart and lungs. It gives an indirect reading of left atrial pressures. The Swan-Ganz catheter is effective for helping to identify structural problems of the heart, such as heart valve or lung disease, that may limit the amount of blood flowing through the heart.

■ OROGASTRIC/NASOGASTRIC TUBE

Orogastric and nasogastric (OG/NG) tubes (Figure 13.5) are inserted into either the mouth or nose (as the names suggest) down into the stomach. They can be used for administration of tube feedings or medications or, more typically in the ICU setting, for decompression of the stomach and removal of gastric contents. Any intubated patient typically has one of these tubes hooked up to low intermittent wall suction to prevent gastric contents from entering the lungs, hopefully preventing aspiration pneumonia. Continuous or high suction settings should be

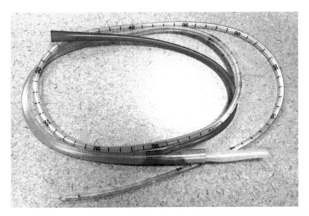

FIGURE 13.5 Orogastric/nasogastric tube. (Photo used with permission from Amalia Cochran, MD, University of Utah.)

avoided because they essentially leave a hickey on the inside of your patient's stomach that may bleed from the irritation. Placement of these tubes can be checked by inserting about 30 mL of air quickly into the tube via syringe while simultaneously listening over the stomach for a telltale gurgle sound. X-ray can also confirm tube placement. Watch for changes to tidal volumes on the ventilator or decreases in oxygen saturation as possible signs that the tube is not in the stomach but is instead in your patient's lungs on an intubated patient. Awake patients typically hate having these inserted but recover quickly once it is in.

◼ DOBHOFF TUBE (ENTERIC FEEDING TUBE)

A Dobhoff tube (DHT) (Figure 13.6) is a tube that is inserted typically through the nose into the stomach or preferentially into the small bowel. It is a small, flexible tube that can remain in for many weeks or months at minimal discomfort to a patient. The purpose of this tube is to provide enteral feeding to a patient for nutrition and for prevention of translocation of gut bacteria. Oral medications can be delivered down a DHT in liquid form or crushed pills. Ideal placement for enteral feeding via DHT is in the duodenum, somewhere past the pyloric sphincter but before the ligament of Treitz to prevent aspiration of tube feeds. Confirmation of placement of this tube can be done with x-ray or with a nifty bedside device that uses radiofrequency that can preclude the need for x-ray.

◼ PERCUTANEOUS ENDOSCOPIC GASTROSTOMY AND PERCUTANEOUS ENDOSCOPIC JEJUNOSTOMY TUBES

A percutaneous endoscopic gastrostomy (PEG) or percutaneous endoscopic jejunostomy (PEJ) tube is placed in a patient who has long-term nutritional needs and is unable to orally consume needed calories and medications. Liquid nutrition and medications can be provided to the patient through the tube. A PEG is a tube that

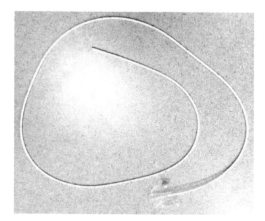

FIGURE 13.6 Nasoenteric feeding tube. (Photo used with permission from Amalia Cochran, MD, University of Utah.)

is placed through the patient's abdominal wall and terminates in the stomach. A PEJ tube is also placed through the abdominal wall and terminates in the jejunum; a PEJ may be used in a patient who has gastric motility issues, a gastric obstruction, or has had their stomach removed.

■ FECAL MANAGEMENT SYSTEM

A fecal management system (FMS) (Figures 13.7–13.8) may also be referred to as a rectal tube. When a patient is incontinent, critically ill, or has a large wound in the perianal area, an FMS is a good tool for keeping liquid stool contained. After it is inserted, a balloon is inflated with a small amount of water to keep the balloon inside the rectum. These tubes can be flushed and repositioned to troubleshoot if they are not draining properly. They need to be removed and the site evaluated every 30 days or they can damage the rectal mucosa.

■ URINARY/FOLEY CATHETER

A Foley catheter (Figure 13.9) is used to drain urine from the bladder. A silicone tube is inserted using aseptic technique into the urethra and travels up to the bladder. A balloon at the distal end of the tube is inflated with sterile saline once it is placed in the bladder, securing it in place. Foleys are placed to prevent wound contamination, to keep the bladder decompressed, and to help monitor a patient's fluid status and kidney perfusion. A "straight" catheter can be used for intermittent drainage of the bladder and is not left in place.

■ CHEST TUBE

A chest tube (Figure 13.10) is inserted to drain air or fluid from the pleural space and is commonly seen in the operating room. The space between the lungs and the ribs can absorb limited amounts of air and fluid, but if too much of either

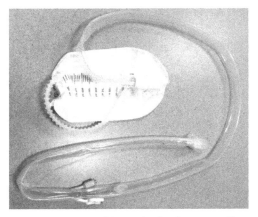

FIGURE 13.7 Fecal management system tubing and collection system Photo used with permission from Amalia Cochran, MD, University of Utah.)

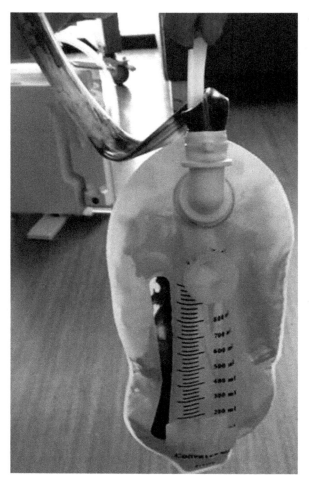

FIGURE 13.8 Fecal management system collection system. (Photo used with permission from Amalia Cochran, MD, University of Utah.)

accumulates, the ability of the lung to function is impaired. Chest tubes can be inserted emergently or intraoperatively as a preventative measure. The tube is inserted into the pleural space and then connected to a chest drainage unit. The chest drainage unit is placed below the patient's chest and maintains negative pressure through suction or water seal. The chest tube drainage unit allows the fluid to be collected and monitored for color and quantity.

■ SURGICAL DRAINS

Surgical drains are used to prevent fluid, such as blood or serous drainage, from accumulating in a surgical incision. Fluid must not sit stagnant in the wound, as it provides a medium for bacteria to grow. Accumulation of excess fluid also affects surrounding organ function.

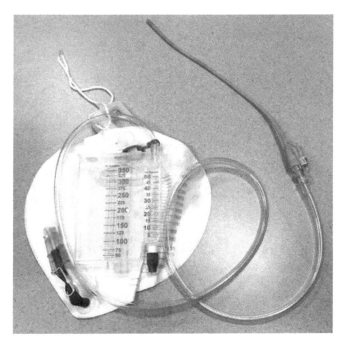

FIGURE 13.9 Foley catheter. (Photo used with permission from Amalia Cochran, MD, University of Utah.)

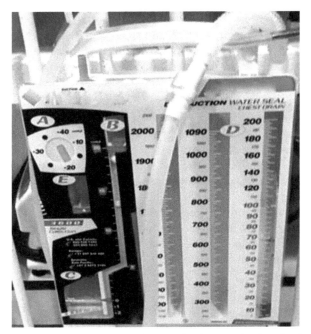

FIGURE 13.10 Chest tube collection system. (Photo used with permission from Amalia Cochran, MD, University of Utah.)

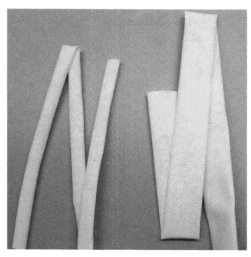

FIGURE 13.11 Penrose drain. (Photo used with permission from Ruth Braga, University of Utah.)

Penrose Drain Open Drainage System

A Penrose drain (Figure 13.11) is a soft, flexible piece of rubber that is placed into a wound. A safety pin is usually pinned at the outermost aspect of the tube to prevent it from sliding into the wound. A piece of fenestrated gauze is placed over the top of the incision with the tube coming out. A second piece of gauze is placed over the top and secured in place with tape. The dressing needs to be changed at least twice a day. The quantity, color, and smell of the drainage is important to document in order to determine wound healing and presence of infection. The Penrose train is considered an "open" drainage system, meaning the fluid is not collected in a sealed container.

Jackson-Pratt and Hemovac Closed Drainage Systems

A closed drainage system uses low negative pressure to eliminate fluid from a surgical site. One end of the drainage tube is placed in the wound and sutured in place where it exits the skin, and the other end is connected to a plastic bulb or container outside the body. The negative pressure created by the compressed bulb or spring-loaded container helps to gently draw fluid from the incision site. The container has a port that allows it to be emptied and retain the negative suction pressure, creating an environment to enhance wound healing. The Jackson-Pratt bulb has a reservoir that will hold about 100 mL of fluid. The Hemovac (Figure 13.12) is used when a larger amount of fluid is expected to be collected, and will hold roughly 400 mL of fluid.

■ NEGATIVE PRESSURE WOUND THERAPY

A negative pressure wound therapy (NPWT) device (Figures 13.13 and 13.14) uses negative pressure to promote vascularization and subsequent granulation

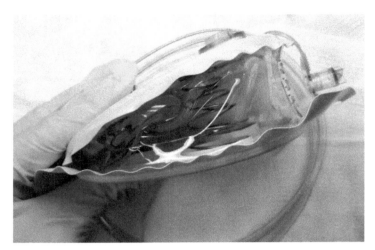

FIGURE 13.12 Hemovac drain. (Photo used with permission from Ruth Braga, University of Utah.)

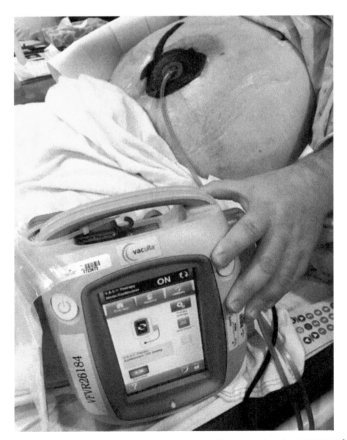

FIGURE 13.13 Negative pressure wound therapy device. (Photo used with permission from Amalia Cochran, University of Utah.)

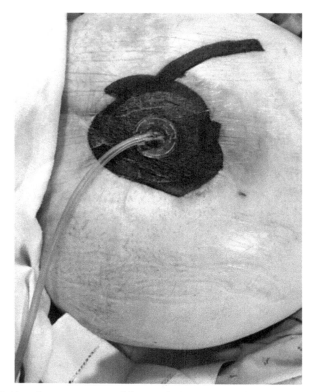

FIGURE 13.14 Negative pressure wound therapy device on a wound. (Photo used with permission from Amalia Cochran, University of Utah.)

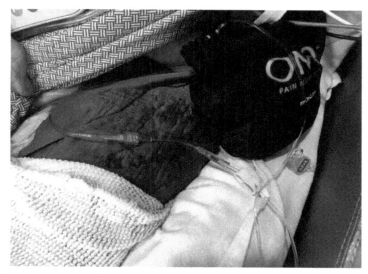

FIGURE 13.15 ON-Q system for continuous infusion of local anesthetic. (Photo used with permission from Amalia Cochran, MD, University of Utah.)

tissue formation for wound healing. NPWT is often used in large open areas that would otherwise provide a wound healing challenge because of either size or location. The wound bed is filled with a sponge-like material. Adhesive tape covers the top of the sponge and is secured to the skin. A small hole is cut in the adhesive tape and a drainage tube is placed on the hole and secured with additional adhesive tape. The drainage tube is connected to a canister that is placed on the NPWT machine. The electrically powered machine applies suction at a set pressure, thus removing drainage and stimulating wound healing. If adequate seal is not maintained the machine will alarm, indicating a leak in the system.

■ ON-Q

ON-Q pumps (Figure 13.15) administer a slow, steady dose of subcutaneously injected analgesia medication for several days following an operation. An ON-Q is a rigid ball that contains the analgesic medication—usually a long-acting local anesthetic—and a small bore catheter delivers the medication. Monitoring an ON-Q can be confusing because they don't deflate over time, so you cannot use the size of the ball to determine how much medication is left in it.

CHAPTER 14

Positioning the Patient

• *Karen Porter, BSN, RN*

Positioning a patient for surgery is much more intricate than you might think (Figures 14.14-14.17). The following series of steps must occur.

◼ STEP 1: TRANSFERRING THE PATIENT TO THE OR TABLE

In order to transfer the patient from their bed to the OR table, both beds are pushed together and locked in place. The surgical team works together to safely transfer the patient, usually with a basic roller board. The surgeon and/or resident and the circulator verify the safety of the patient. The patient is NEVER left unattended through this process, particularly once anesthesia has been induced.

◼ STEP 2: PLACING SEQUENTIAL COMPRESSION DEVICES (SCDS) TO THE PATIENT'S LEGS

These leg-warmer-like wraps are wound around the patient's legs, secured, and connected to a machine that creates a squeezing action on each leg. The squeezing action of the SCDs assists with blood flow and prevents blood clots. This is a priority action for patient safety and they must be on prior to anesthesia induction.

◼ STEP 3: POSITIONING OF THE ASLEEP PATIENT

Many basic positions exist for patient positioning for operative cases. Some of the most common are supine, prone, low lithotomy, and lateral decubitus. Correct positioning of the patient is one of the basic essential functions of every case. It can be done well when the OR team works together to ensure the safety of the patient. The patient is positioned in the most anatomically appropriate position for the surgery, safety straps are applied, pressure points are padded, and genitals are checked. Padding and positioning can be enhanced by the use of gel pads, pillows, foam pads, blanket rolls … there are numerous options. Anesthesia verifies that the head and neck are in correct alignment and that there are no pressure points on the face or neck. The patient's ultimate position depends on what needs to be done, but access to the surgical site and comfort/safety of the patient are paramount. Because the patient is unable to move during surgery, it is critical that we check for potential circulatory, musculoskeletal, and neurological injuries that could occur. The ultimate goal is to have no postoperative injuries or complications due to positioning.

■ STEP 4: MOVING THE FURNITURE AROUND

During surgery the OR table height is often changed. When the height of the table goes up, the mayo stand needs to go up so it doesn't place pressure on the patient's feet. Anesthesia communicates this to the team and the scrub tech will adjust the mayo. They might ask you to move your arms so they can move the tray. Please remember that while you may rest your hands on the patient if you are scrubbed, you must be mindful of leaning on the patient—particularly if they are a very small patient. A small amount of your weight can really impact a pediatric patient's physiology.

■ STEP 5: WHAT HAPPENS AT THE END

Just as it took a village to get the patient properly positioned on the OR table, the same process must occur in reverse to get them back to their patient bed. The patient's safety remains all of our responsibility during this transfer, particularly because they will often still be under general anesthesia. Also, we need to assess the condition of the patient's skin and document this assessment. Hopefully other than the surgical site it is intact and in the same condition as when the patient came in. If not, the surgeon needs to be made aware, the condition should be passed along in report, and an incident report should be filed.

■ AN EXERCISE

Think about your posture right now. How are your arms hanging? Are your palms facing out? No. Rotate them out and keep them there for a few moments. Is that comfortable for you? Probably not. How about after a 4-hour surgery? As a newcomer to the OR, now is the time to be paying attention and learning these basic skills. Think about finishing a long, complicated case. From a surgical standpoint it went smoothly. You don't want the patient to develop a pressure sore due to lack of padding or a nerve injury because someone incorrectly positioned the patient's hands. The preparations made for surgery can be just as important as the surgery itself.

A few of the positions and equipment that are used in the OR are listed here.

Bed remote. Looking at the bed remote (Figure 14.1), you can see just how many positions there are.

Operating rooms have closets filled with thousands of materials, nuts and bolts, pads, and items to position patients (Figures 14.2–14.5).

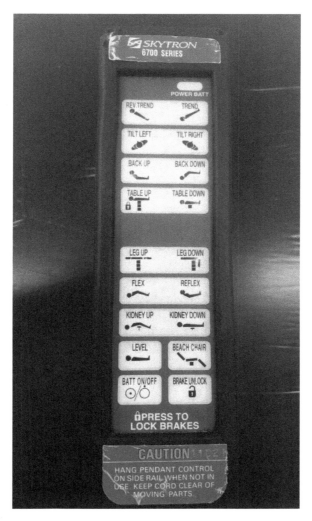

FIGURE 14.1 The remote to control the OR bed. (Photo used with permission from Karen Porter, University of Utah.)

Although the OR beds are soft, they are not soft enough for comfort for hours at a time. Gel padding (Figure 14.6) is added to supplement and pad bony prominences. It can easily be wiped off and cleaned for the next patient.

Sequential compression devices (Figures 14.7 and 14.8) must not only be on the patient, but attached to the machine and plugged in.

Supine position (Figures 14.9 and 14.10) is one of the most common positions in general surgery. Arms are extended in a natural position, elbows are padded, and arms are loosely strapped on to ensure that they don't flop off. A pillow is

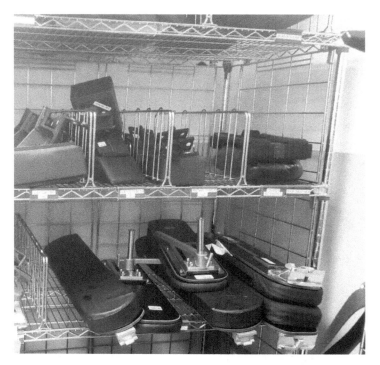

FIGURE 14.2 A collection of arm boards and other pads and supports. (Photo used with permission from Karen Porter, University of Utah.)

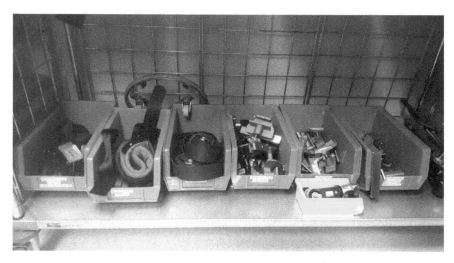

FIGURE 14.3 Straps and brackets for the OR table. (Photo used with permission from Karen Porter, University of Utah.)

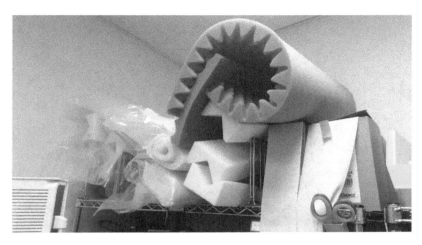

FIGURE 14.4 "Egg crates" and other pads for patient positioning. (Photo used with permission from Karen Porter, University of Utah.)

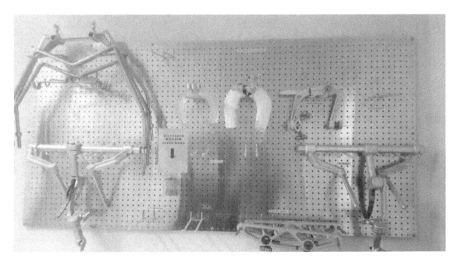

FIGURE 14.5 The "Mayfield," used for craniotomy positioning. (Photo used with permission from Karen Porter, University of Utah.)

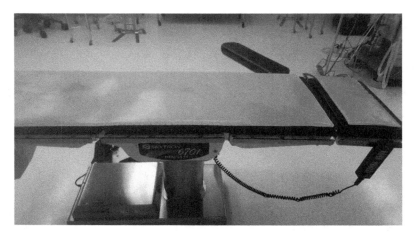

FIGURE 14.6 Gel pad placed on an OR table. (Photo used with permission from Karen Porter, University of Utah.)

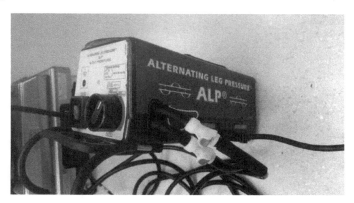

FIGURE 14.7 A sequential compression device (SCD) machine. (Photo used with permission from Ruth Braga, University of Utah.)

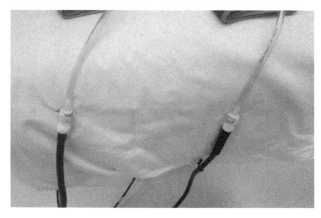

FIGURE 14.8 SCD tubing. (Photo used with permission from Karen Porter, University of Utah.)

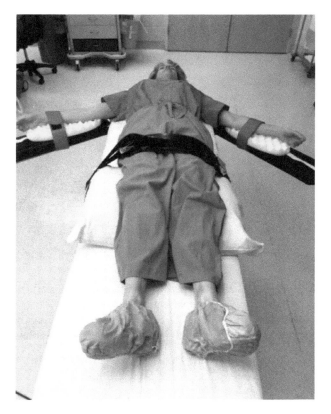

FIGURE 14.9 Supine patient positioned with arms out on the OR table. (Photo used with permission from Ruth Braga, University of Utah.)

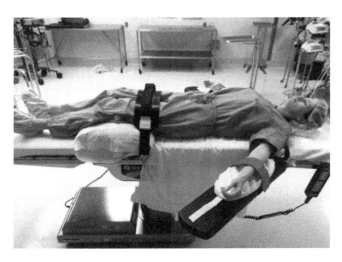

FIGURE 14.10 Side view of a safely padded and positioned supine patient on the OR table. (Photo used with permission from Ruth Braga, University of Utah.)

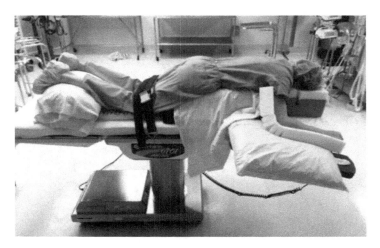

FIGURE 14.11 Safely padded and positioned prone patient. (Photo used with permission from Ruth Braga, University of Utah.)

placed under the knees to alleviate pressure on the back. A padded safety strap goes across the thighs, securing the patient to the OR bed.

Prone position (Figures 14.11 and 14.12): anesthesia controls the padding of the face into a specialized pillow which keeps the endotracheal tube from putting

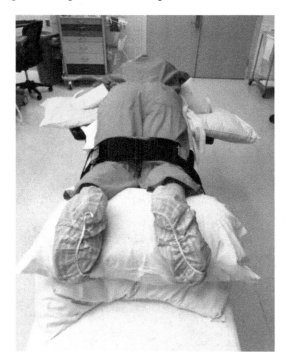

FIGURE 14.12 Positioning of the feet/toes for a prone patient. (Photo used with permission from Ruth Braga, University of Utah.)

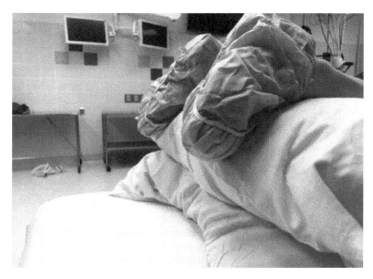

FIGURE 14.13 Side view of foot positioning for a prone patient. (Photo used with permission from Ruth Braga, University of Utah.)

pressure on the face. The knees, abdomen, and elbows are padded and positioned as naturally as possible. We always check to make sure that toes are hanging freely (Figure 14.13), and that weight is distributed evenly.

Padded elbows and hands (Figures 14.14 and 14.15). There are a variety of specialized pieces of padding such as the face pillow and specially formed elbow pads. Whether it is a specialty item or a plain pillow, we always double-check that the

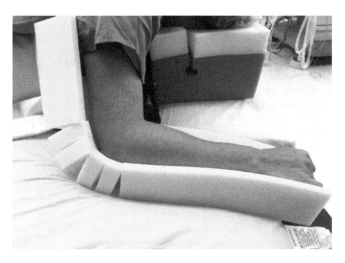

FIGURE 14.14 Padded elbows in a prone patient. (Photo used with permission from Karen Porter, University of Utah.)

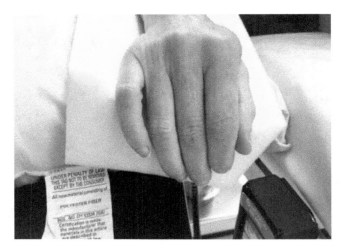

FIGURE 14.15 Padded hand/fingers. (Photo used with permission from Ruth Braga, University of Utah.)

body is in as natural a position as possible. Safe positioning takes the hands and eyes of many, walking around the patient and checking everything.

Lateral position (Figure 14.16) takes an even greater amount of teamwork, effort, and double-checking. Because lying on your side for even a small amount of time can be uncomfortable, it is crucial that we are certain our patient is properly positioned.

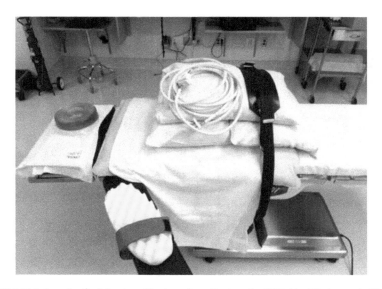

FIGURE 14.16 Supplies for lateral positioning of a patient on the OR table. (Photo used with permission from Karen Porter, University of Utah.)

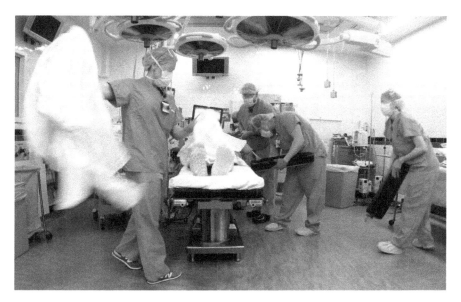

FIGURE 14.17 Team working together to position the patient on the OR table. (Photo used with permission from Ruth Braga, University of Utah.)

It takes a team (Figure 14.17). For some complex cases, proper positioning can take 15 minutes or longer. It takes everyone who is available to ensure that the patient is safe and positioned as optimally as possible for the surgeon to be able to access the site.

CHAPTER 15

Patient Safety in the OR

• *Jon Worthen, MSN, RN, CNOR*

"Welcome to the OR!" is not the initial greeting you are likely to hear on your first day in the OR. "Whoa there!" is typically the first salutation you'll receive if you get too close to the sterile field. More than likely you'll think you are at a rodeo, not because we use stirrups but because things happen fast. *Controlled chaos* is among the terms used by those observing in the OR for the first time. One of the things as educator and circulator I emphasize while orienting new RNs, medical students, and OR first-timers is that our first concern is always patient safety.

Envision for a moment the OR from the patient's perspective. The patient makes an appointment with their primary care provider (PCP) for either a routine physical or if something unusual is happening—pain, a lump, or an "unusual" feeling. Typically, they have an extended relationship with this provider where trust has already been established. The PCP then refers the patient to a surgeon with whom the patient meets once (that's plenty of time to build an extensive relationship of trust, right?). Then, the next thing they know they are in the a.m. admission or same-day surgery (SDS) unit getting ready for surgery. The SDS RN then calls the OR RN for handoff communication. This is a safety briefing, ensuring that pertinent information is passed along to each caregiver. This is usually done in an SBAR (situation, background, assessment, recommendations) format. This gives us an organized format to deliver a brief and appropriately detailed report specific to the patient and allows the OR RN to plan for the specific needs of the patient.

Next, the patient is in route to the OR and they have had nothing to eat or drink since midnight. They're nervous and hungry, which can translate into lightheadedness and dizziness. In addition, an IV has just been started before they were transferred to the OR. What does this equate to? Fall risk. All of our patients in the perioperative setting are at risk for falls. As our patients proceed to the OR, we talk to them in a preoperative holding area, and inevitably most need to go to the bathroom one more time—they will need an escort to the bathroom.

Bathroom duties handled, they are back on the gurney and headed to the OR suite. However, they stop first at the "red line" (Figure 15.1). "Red line," you ask? That's what designates the need for OR attire beyond the line. It's one of our steps in keeping the patient safe.

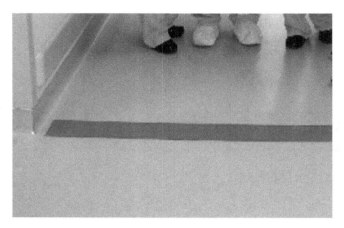

FIGURE 15.1 The infamous "red line" that you must be in OR attire to cross. (Photo used with permission from Ruth Braga, University of Utah.)

Now for my soapbox. OR attire is there for a reason, so if you are an MD, med student, PA, NP, RN or anyone else, let's be clear: OR attire is just that—attire for the operating room (Figure 15.2). If I wear my scrubs home, yes, I may look cool as I stop at the grocery store on the way home but I've just been in a bloody, contaminated OR. Then I am going home and throwing my scrubs in with my family's laundry (that's a pleasant thought). Then we take those "clean" scrubs and wear them from home where I have just been playing with my dog and proceed to the OR. Get it? Change your scrubs at the hospital. Patient safety starts with you.

Okay, now I'm getting off of my soapbox and heading back to the red line. This is also where the patient struggles emotionally. They lose their support system. This where they are separated from their families, so sensitivity is crucial. The OR crew needs to fill this gap and build trust in a short period of time. Explaining to the patient what is happening and what is going to happen can ease their anxiety and that of their family. This is a great time to allow the patient to voice any concerns or questions they may have.

Rolling into the OR, the patient may be given medication to help them relax. Three to four members of the surgical team need to surround them and assist the patient in moving to the OR bed. If you are new to the OR and have any patient care experience, you may be asked to assist. Be sure you clearly understand what you are being asked to do. A circulator, scrub, anesthesiologist, and surgeon would much rather clarify a sentence or two than have an injury due to a communication error. So, bottom line ... if you're not sure, ask. You'll also gain the crew's respect much faster. There is nothing that will destroy trust more quickly than a new person in the OR faking it. We can tell. Remember, we all had to learn this whole new environment at some time. It is a phenomenal place where our patients place a vast amount of trust in us. Take time to ask. That keeps you, your team members, and the patient safe.

The next thing you will observe is a safety strap placed on the patient (Figure 15.3). Our beds are narrow and sudden moves of an unrestrained patient

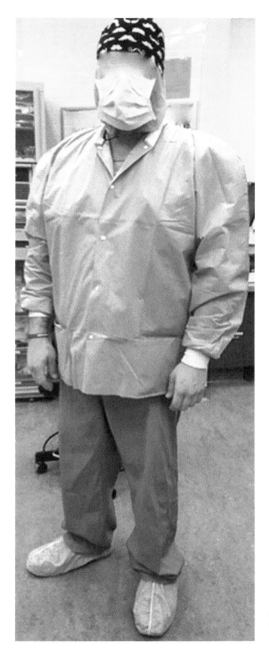

FIGURE 15.2 Appropriate OR attire (although some institutions do not allow custom scrub caps). (Photo used with permission from Ruth Braga, University of Utah.)

can be catastrophic. The RN will be at the side of the patient as the patient drifts off to sleep. While the airway is being established for intubation, this is where the anesthesiologist and circulating RN need to be focused. If they don't answer your questions immediately during this stage of the surgery, that need for focus

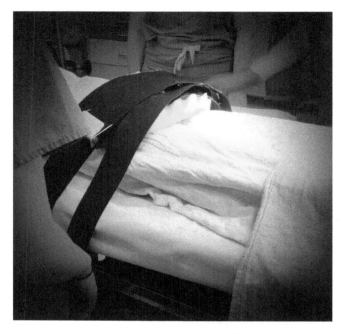

FIGURE 15.3 Padding the patient and placing the safety belt. (Photo used with permission from Ruth Braga, University of Utah.)

is the reason. Once the airway is secured, the patient is positioned. Again, it takes multiple hands to keep the patient steady and position them correctly. Orderlies or other staff members are usually there to assist. Specialized devices are used for each position to keep the patient safe and prevent any nerve damage, pressure injuries, or other complications. You'll see the circulator or other members of the team meticulously position the patient to ensure safety. When training new nurses, I would commonly gather them in an OR not being used and have them try positioning each other so they could see and feel the different pressure points that occur in different positions.

After positioning the patient, we prep, drape, and do a final time-out verification. This is to ensure patient safety by identifying that we are performing the correct procedure on the correct patient. Prior to incision, a sponge, sharps, and instrument count must be completed. What goes into the patient must come out. We track this count on a white board in the room.

Sharps safety is paramount. I've witnessed OR crewmembers cut with scalpels, drill bits, rake retractors, sharp towel clips, and a host of other surgical tools. Puncture wounds can also occur in different situations such as while passing a needle holder with loaded suture, while closing an incision, or when the needle is resting on the mayo stand or back table. If you get to scrub in, be sharps aware. It is best to keep your hands away from the mayo stand (the main little table over the patient where the most immediate needed instruments are kept). If you're not scrubbed

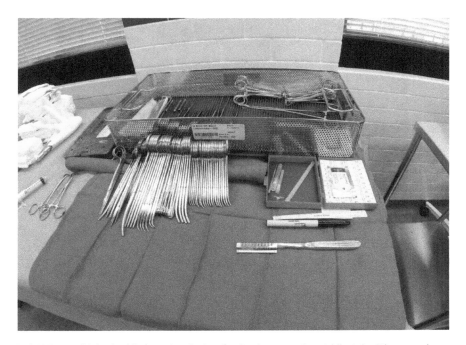

FIGURE 15.4 OR back table featuring the box for the sharps on the middle right. (Photo used with permission from Ruth Braga, University of Utah.)

in, let the tech or the RN handle the sharps at the end of the case. It's great to offer to help, but let them take care of the sharps (Figure 15.4).

While you are in the OR, the experience is fascinating. It is so incredible to witness firsthand how harmoniously the different systems of the body work (Figure 15.5). We can get so caught up in the moment that sometimes we forget about OR safety for ourselves. In addition to sharps, various equipment, cords, or IV lines can also create hazards for staff or visitors (Figure 15.6). Additionally, if you are involved in an arthroscopic case that uses liter upon liter of fluid to irrigate the joint, OR puddles and even lakes may form that would make drought-stricken areas in California envious. These, combined with the smooth OR floors, can be treacherous. Be vigilant of these hazards and move slowly and deliberately when navigating a wet OR floor.

Hazards with equipment exist as well. Electrocautery is used in the OR to help control bleeding with electrical current. A grounding pad is used to keep the patient safe. However, I have seen a team member jump from minor electric shock because of an unnoticed hole in their glove while cauterizing. Cautery, if not managed correctly, can also cause injury to the patient (Figure 15.7). Cautery and wet preps don't mix. You'll often hear the circulator let the surgeon know when the prep is dry. Prep solutions containing alcohol need to dry completely before draping. If the prep site is still wet when draping, the alcohol may not dry and electrocautery can inflame a situation, literally. OR fires can begin when the alcohol in the prep solution is ignited by the cautery. This is an extremely dangerous situation

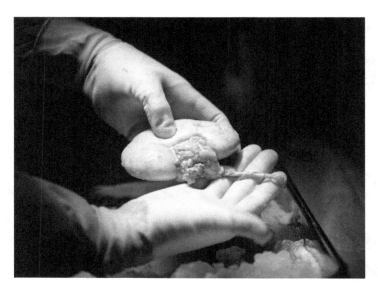

FIGURE 15.5 Explanted kidney, ready for transplantation. (Photo used with permission from Transplant Service, University of Utah).

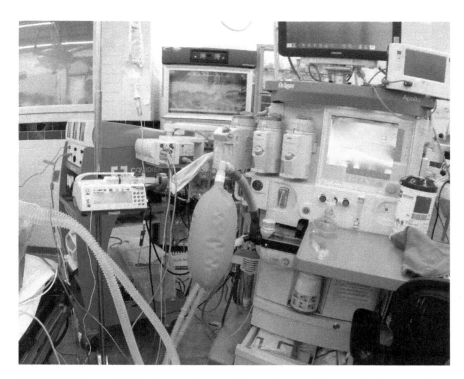

FIGURE 15.6 Beware all of the lines and tubes as tripping hazards. (Photo used with permission from Ruth Braga, University of Utah.)

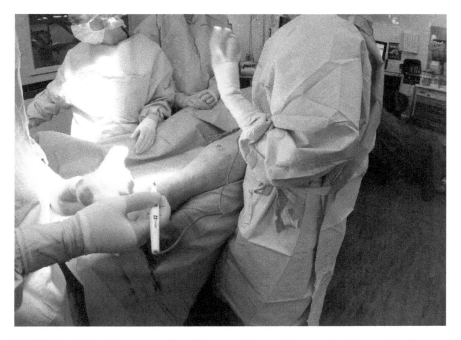

FIGURE 15.7 Bovie electrocautery "pencil" prepared for use. (Photo used with permission from Ruth Braga, University of Utah.)

that can have catastrophic outcomes. A quick response is necessary to contain the fire. Other ignition sources include the intense light sources for arthroscopic and laparoscopic procedures. These light sources attach to the scope to be used internally, but if detached from the scope and placed on a sponge or a drape can quickly start a fire. Lasers are another source of danger. Intense beams from the lasers can accidently start fires if unintentionally activated. Foot pedals activate some laser and electrocautery units. So be sure to watch your step and think about things that might be flammable.

So now it's the end of the procedure and time to move the patient safely to the gurney or bed. The OR RN and anesthesiologist will give a handoff report to the receiving nurse. The patient did well and you survived. You wore proper attire, helped them cope emotionally, did not allow the patient to fall, clarified and communicated your questions. You observed the time-out, didn't get stuck with a needle, and did not fall amidst the various equipment and swamps. You watched the prep dry and didn't rest your foot on a cautery foot pedal … no OR fire here. The most excellent thing of all, you witnessed the miraculous workings of the human body and were able to participate in the finest department … the best kept secret in healthcare—working in the OR. Congratulations to you!

CHAPTER 16

Distractions and Interruptions in the Operating Room

• *Nick Sevdalis, PhD and Louise Hull, PhD*

Think about the last time you were at home, relaxed on the sofa, completely immersed in a film. The lights are low, you feel the tension building—you're trying to figure out what will happen next. Then one of your roommates bursts into the room and turns all the lights on. She is upset, she failed an exam. You feel for her, stop the film and spend the next 10 minutes consoling her. You're grateful when she leaves and allows you to go back to the film. A few minutes later, your phone rings—you reject the call, but it rings again. One of your medical schoolmates wants to talk to you; he's in trouble with his girlfriend (again…). As a Good Samaritan, you lend him a sympathetic ear for a few minutes. When he is calmer, he gets off the phone and you're once again free to enjoy the film. But a few minutes later your other roommates arrive home—will you help to carry the groceries from the car? asks one. Of course you will. As you bring the last bag to the kitchen they ask you to join them for dinner—after all, you haven't seen them much lately. You accept, as you don't want to be the only one not joining in, but by now you're in a rather foul mood—and the rest of the movie will have to wait.

Now, let's put this scenario aside—and let's think of being in the operating room (OR), repairing a right inguinal hernia of a 77-year-old overweight male patient with medically controlled angina and diabetes. Your attending is assisting you actively because you're early on in your learning curve, not having done many of these. You're a junior resident; you're keen to get your numbers up and impress the seniors. Unfortunately, you can't quite focus. Since the beginning of the procedure there have been problems with the OR list—there has been an error, apparently, as the first patient should have been last on the list (she has latex allergy) but no one seemed to know about it. The OR chief nurse is very irritated and so is the attending anesthesiologist—the start of the list has been delayed and now you're running late. Various people, many of whom you have never seen before, have been in and out of the OR to confer with the team, and your attending manages most of this while you're trying to focus on the case. There is a radio playing in the background, and someone has left their pager on a stool on the side of the room; the pager goes off every few minutes. At the point when you're trying to cut the mesh to the right size, a rather angry OR suite manager walks into the room to say that the next case will now have to be cancelled and put on the next available slot. Now your attending gets angry, as he is about to go on holiday and this will clearly mess things up. A heated conversation ensues—you're keeping your head down and trying to take the case forward, but your boss eventually takes over to speed things up. The next patient is brought into the OR suite shortly after this case is completed. The patient is rolled onto the operating table as you're writing up the notes for the previous case and the next thing you hear is the senior OR nurse yelling at the anesthesiologist that this patient is the one with the latex allergy, who somehow was brought forward on the list. You sigh. The chaos will clearly continue throughout the day (Figure 16.1).

What does watching a movie at home have in common with repairing a hernia in the OR? In both of these examples, people were initially engrossed in a task (watching a movie, doing a procedure), and then distracted from it multiple times. The outcome is negative in both cases—irritability with a ruined evening in the first case, an avoidable error in dealing with an allergic patient in the second. Being distracted while doing something enjoyable or while completing a complex task is a well-documented phenomenon, and both of the examples above are real. In fact, distractions and interruptions are pretty much part of real life. How often are we

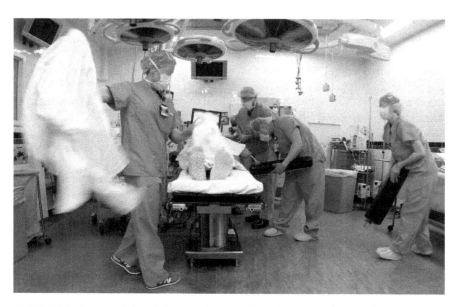

FIGURE 16.1 "Organized chaos" often describes the OR environment. (Photo used with permission from Ruth Braga, University of Utah.)

able to achieve the level of focus and concentration we need to do a job to the best of our ability, or to enjoy a sport or hobby fully? The modern world keeps adding distractions to our lives. Numerous recent studies document the abundance of stimulation in our environment, much of which is electronic in the form of social media and smart phone applications. Distractions and interruptions in our lives engender the phenomenon of multitasking—trying to do more than one thing simultaneously. Think of drivers listening to the news on the radio while simultaneously having a conversation with the person sitting next to them, while they try to take a call on their cell phone. This is a classic example of multitasking.

Although ubiquitous in our lives, doing more than one thing at the same time is not usually ideal. Psychologists have spent years examining what happens to our performance when we multitask. In these studies, a main task is typically designated (e.g., watch a movie, repair a hernia, or drive a car), along with a secondary task (e.g., help a friend, manage a list, or talk to the car passenger). The evidence tends to show that we get worse outcomes at the main task when we multitask—when distractors are added into the mix. Simply put, we're normally better off watching a movie, repairing someone's hernia, or driving home without being interrupted (or interrupting ourselves) with other tasks. Another key finding is that our ability to manage distractions and multitask effectively is variable. Higher levels of expertise in skilled tasks typically mean we are better able to cope with distractions; also, less demanding distractions cause less of a detriment to our performance. There are also individual differences in our innate ability and desire to multitask.

How frequently does an OR team get distracted while doing a case? While will vary from one OR to another, observational studies in the OR have showed that distractions occur disturbingly often—for example, every 2 or every 10 minutes. Distractions also affect the perioperative pathway—when the patient is being put to sleep, during the procedure, and while the patient is being awakened for transfer to the recovery room. This means that all OR team members are affected by distractions. The OR is not alone in this, as distractions have been identified in emergency departments (where they abound), hospital wards, and community-based primary care practices.

It thus appears that healthcare delivery is riddled with distractions—but does it matter? After all, most of us are able to drive a car while talking to the person sitting next to us. The short answer to the question is yes, distractions do matter, as they affect care negatively. They predispose individuals and teams to errors because they are linked to lack of safety checks throughout procedures in the OR and higher rates of surgical site infection. The problem we have is that often an individual does not realize they are being distracted until it is too late; for example, in the case of driving, when an accident occurs. As a result of studies on drivers, many countries have laws that drivers cannot hold a mobile phone and talk while driving, to minimize this impact. In commercial aviation, there is the concept of "sterile cockpit," which means that at safety-critical phases of a flight no irrelevant communications are allowed within the cockpit, in order to maintain pilot focus and reduce the risk of human error due to distraction or interruption.

Interestingly, there are some tasks where an element of periodic distraction may be useful. Such tasks typically involve monitoring, which humans are not very good at. Monitoring is what happens in large control rooms of industrial plants, or is what anesthesiologists often have to do for prolonged periods of time during a case. Looking at a screen for hours on end is not the most captivating activity and in such activities levels of concentration may drop off over time. One way to address this problem is by introducing some distraction every now and then to alleviate boredom (Figure 16.2).

The evidence base is still developing—but overall we seem to be heading in a similar direction as other industries that have established that distractions are detrimental when handling cars or planes. A PubMed search on distractions or interruptions will reveal many interesting studies—including one that found different effects of music on laparoscopic task dexterity when the participants liked or disliked the music they were listening to. Most of the studies done in ORs are observational, but many other studies of distractions are performed in simulated environments. It would be neither ethical nor desirable to randomize patients to pleasant or unpleasant distracting music and then measure the effect on the surgeon's dexterity.

So what is the take-home message? Distractors will lower performance and concentration in the OR when you're operating, especially during your early, formative years. You should actively manage them by not tolerating an environment that makes you (and your colleagues, whether they realize it or not) more prone to lapses in concentration resulting in errors. Establishing some basic and simple rules in the OR, like a "sterile OR" when doing complex dissection or at safety-critical phases of a procedure, is a sign of maturity and safety consciousness that will benefit both you and your patients.

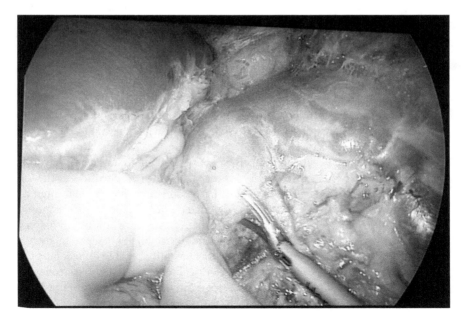

FIGURE 16.2 View of a laparoscopic screen monitor intraoperatively. (Photo used with permission from Charlie Ehlert, University of Utah.)

CHAPTER 17

A View into the Operating Room

• *Ruth Braga, MSN, RN*

The closed doors of the operating room create quite a mystery for those on the outside. To share some insight, we have gathered a variety of photos that show stages of an operation in a few different locations. You will notice many similarities and a few differences—primarily with the supplies used and the table setup. Because devices, techniques, staff, patient needs, and equipment are constantly changing, don't ever expect the time to come when you say, "I have seen it all."

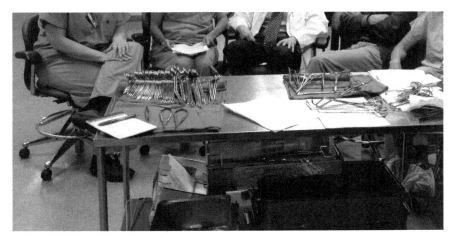

FIGURE 17.1 In-service training on instrumentation with the University of Utah Transplant Team. (Photo used with permission from Transplant Service, University of Utah.)

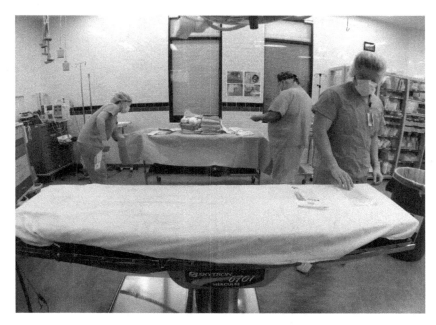

FIGURE 17.2 OR staff preparing the room for the next case. (Photo used with permission from Ruth Braga, University of Utah.)

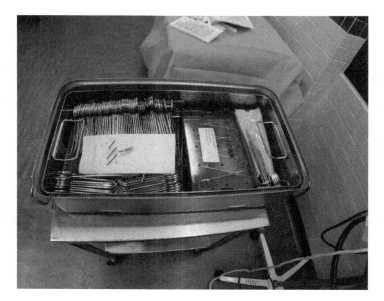

FIGURE 17.3 A freshly opened pan of sterilized instruments. The striped tape indicates that the pan has been properly sterilized. (Photo used with permission from Ruth Braga, University of Utah.)

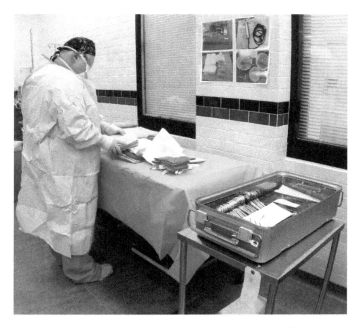

FIGURE 17.4 Gowned and gloved scrub technician preparing his back table for an OR case. (Photo used with permission from Ruth Braga, University of Utah.)

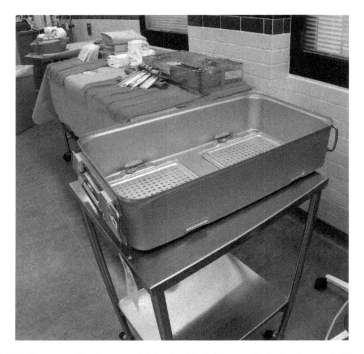

FIGURE 17.5 Empty sterilization pan with back table fully set up in the background. (Photo used with permission from Ruth Braga, University of Utah.)

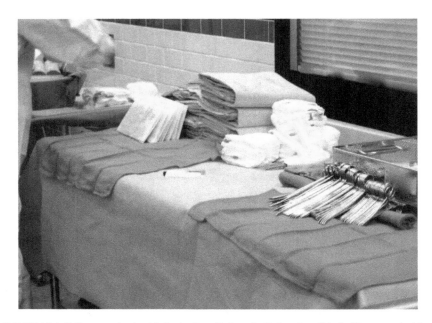

FIGURE 17.6 Fully set up back table in the Burn Unit at the University of Utah. (Photo used with permission from Ruth Braga, University of Utah.)

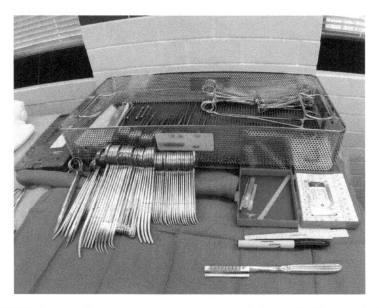

FIGURE 17.7 Close-up of instrument pan contents set up on the back table. (Photo used with permission from Ruth Braga, University of Utah.)

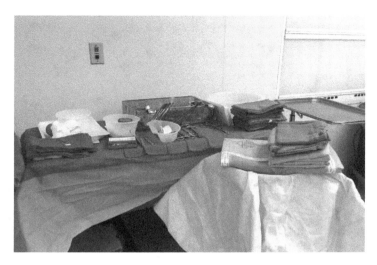

FIGURE 17.8 Fully set up back table at UCLA. (Photo used with permission from Deanna Attai, MD; Geffen School of Medicine at UCLA, UCLA Health Burbank Breast Care.)

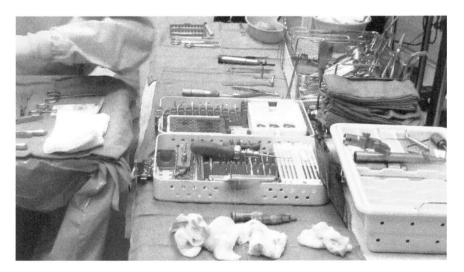

FIGURE 17.9 Orthopedic surgery setup during a case. (Photo used with permission from Ruth Braga, University of Utah.)

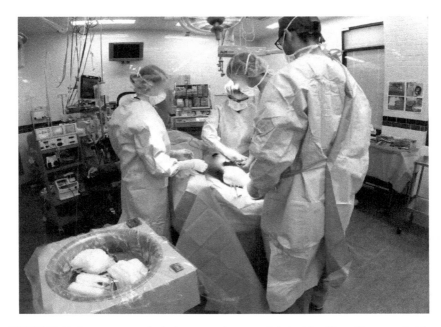

FIGURE 17.10 Surgeons at work placing a tourniquet to minimize blood loss. (Photo used with permission from Ruth Braga, University of Utah.)

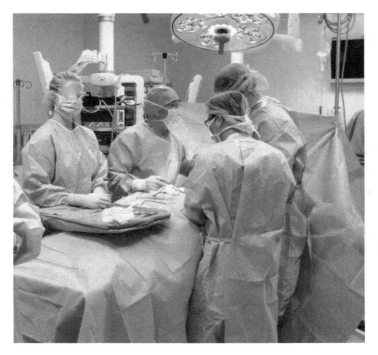

FIGURE 17.11 Dr. McGreevy patiently teaches residents in the operating room. (Photo used with permission from Ruth Braga, University of Utah.)

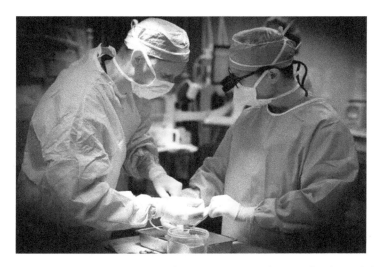

FIGURE 17.12 Surgeons preparing a kidney for transplantation. (Photo used with permission from the Transplant Service, University of Utah.)

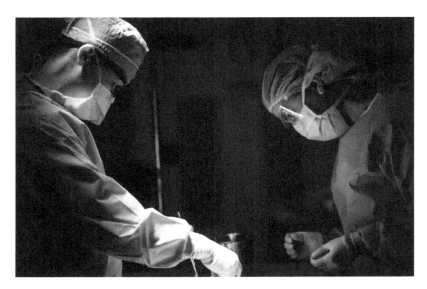

FIGURE 17.13 Surgeons preparing a kidney for transplantation. This preparation takes place at a table right next to where the patient is being operated on. (Photo used with permission from the Transplant Service, University of Utah.)

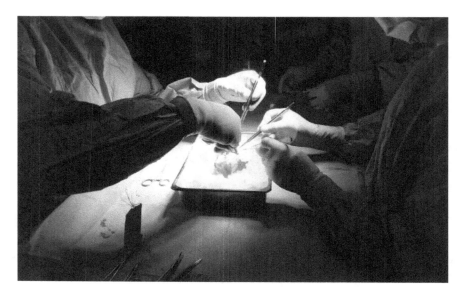

FIGURE 17.14 Up-close view of surgeons preparing a kidney for transplantation. (Photo used with permission from the Transplant Service, University of Utah.)

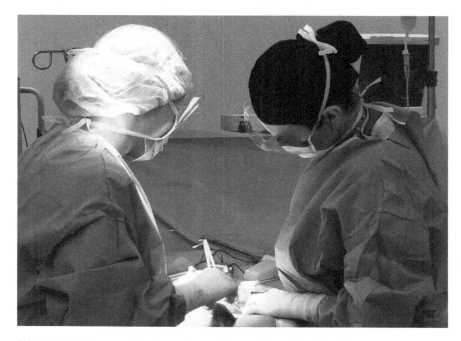

FIGURE 17.15 Intraoperative photo of a surgical attending and resident discussing the next step in a case. (Photo used with permission from Sarah Bryczkowski, MD; Rutgers-UMDNJ Department of Surgery.)

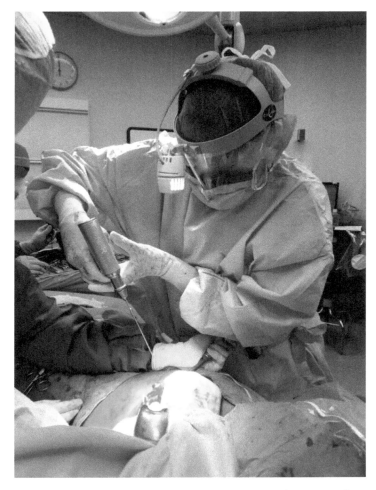

FIGURE 17.16 Intraoperative orthopedic procedeure. (Photo used with permission from Sarah Bryczkowski, MD; Rutgers-UMDNJ Department of Surgery.)

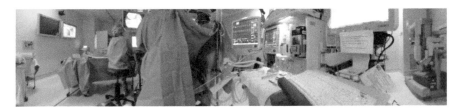

FIGURE17.17 Panoramic view of a "green room" from anesthesia's perspective. (Photo used with permission from J. P. Meizoso, M.D; DeWitt Daughtry Family Department of Surgery University of Miami Miller School of Medicine.)

And Now For More Entertainment…

Notes from Your Attending

• *Lawrence A. Shirley, MD and Christian Jones, MD, FACS*

First time in the OR, huh? Well, don't touch anything. Just put your hands where I tell you to. You're probably not going to understand anything we're doing, so you can ask some questions when it's a good time. As long as you read for the cases, you'll be fine. Sit back and watch the master at work.

Don't mind him. It's easy to lose sight of how overwhelming this place can be. To make things more difficult, every OR is a little bit different. We'll try to give you some tips that will apply to most of them and get you off on the right foot for the others. The first tip, as you've probably already guessed, is that the operating theatre (to use an old-school and Very British term) is a very structured place, with a long list of rules (both published and unpublished), and it can be tense at times. One of the key roles of the attending surgeon (which some fill better than others) is to make sure the right level of tension is maintained; too much tension makes the team ineffective, while too little could lead to distraction.

■ PREP BEFORE OR

All right, so you think you are worthy of attempting to grace the hallowed halls of my operating room? Well, just know that I expect you to know EVERYTHING about the patient we are about to treat. I mean, shoe size, what they had for dinner two weeks ago, great-grandmother's maiden name. EVERYTHING. However, don't talk to me beforehand. Don't make eye contact, as a matter of fact. Speak when spoken to, and softly at that.

Okay, so this is a little extreme, don't you think? It is true: most of us expect you to know as much about the patient as is feasible and appropriate. It is important for you to know why we are taking this particular patient to the OR, why we felt that an operation is what this person needed. Next, read about the operation itself. How is it performed? A brief review of a surgical atlas will help you understand what we are doing, keep you engaged during the surgery by knowing the anatomy and the steps, and will impress the heck out your attending. Know about the disease process that necessitates operative intervention. Know about alternative treatments and possible complications of the procedure. That said, we understand how incredibly hectic and tiring it can be as a medical student on their first surgery rotation. Two or three years ago, you were an undergraduate trying to schedule all of your classes to start no earlier than noon, and now you're waking up at 4 a.m. to be the first to round on patients, and then running from time commitment to time commitment. Maybe you were assigned to scrub the case 5 seconds before its scheduled start time. We remember what it was like. Just try your best. Be interested. Care about learning, care about the patient.

Here is a list of people who work in the perioperative area to whom you should feel comfortable introducing yourself: everyone. When it looks like we, the attendings, are free from distractions, introduce yourself to us. Introduce yourself to the patient and the patient's family if no one from the surgery team has already done so. Explain your role to these people to increase their comfort level. Introduce yourself to the anesthesia team, the peri-operative nursing team, and the OR staff before the case starts. You will be surprised at how quickly you become included as a member of the team by introducing yourself, and by learning other team members' names.

■ WHAT TO DO WHEN THE PATIENT IS GOING TO SLEEP

So, are you just going to stand there? How about a little shave? No, not for me, for the patient—you aren't going to make a cut in that hairy mess are you? Forget it, the nurse can do that. Just get the lights and slam a catheter in. Page me when you're prepped.

Now's a good time to bring up that we have no idea what you know and what you don't. You may have been an emergency department technician before medical school and placed hundreds of nasogastric tubes and urinary catheters. You may, on the other hand, be wondering which tube goes in which hole. Anywhere on that spectrum is just fine as long as you admit where you are. As you've hopefully already discovered, one of the best ways to approach any such task is to admit when you don't know how to do something and ask to learn. "Learning by doing" is great. Learning by faking it and putting a patient at risk isn't. We remember that performing invasive procedures on an awake patient can be mighty intimidating, so now is your chance to learn while the patient is asleep. Don't be afraid to ask if you can learn how to place these tubes and catheters.

Even if you're new to the OR, you can still help get everything prepared and move the preoperative time along. The nurses and technicians have a great deal of work to finish before the first incision, and with much of it you're not allowed to help. However, anyone can help position the patient properly, move the overhead lights so that they're pointing at the area where we'll be operating, help place sequential compression devices, and, once taught, remove any unwanted hair from that area. If you haven't already met the members of the OR team, now's a good time; and if you can't think of anything to do, one of the nicest ways for you to endear yourself to the OR staff is by asking them what you can do to help.

■ HOW TO GET SCRUBBED IN

What exactly are you doing? Did anyone actually teach you how to scrub? Here, just watch me. Wet your hands, rub soap on them with the brush, and then let them dry. Or, I guess, you can use the alcohol thing, but nobody who knows what they're doing really does. How much more difficult could you possibly make it? No, not like that. Okay, now you've got to start over. Do it like I was doing. No, like I was doing. Maybe you should sit this one out and just watch. No, then I'll just get the same evaluations again.... Nurse? Nurse! Can you get out here to show this one how to scrub?

Scrubbing isn't hard, but it's systematic, and there are plenty of little things that mess us up. That's right, we still mess up with something as simple and routine as scrubbing from time to time as well. Before you go to the scrub area, ensure the scrub tech or nurse has sterile gloves and a gown available for you. If you're wearing a ring or a watch, take it off and put it somewhere that you won't lose it or put it into the laundry. Take your pager or phone off and leave them on the counter. Then ensure your mask is just as you like it and your eye protection is in place; once scrubbed, you won't be able to touch them again until the case is done.

Depending on your hospital, people may preferentially use an alcohol-based surgical hand scrub or a traditional wet hand scrub. Either is acceptable but you can learn how to do both in your OR orientation and then use whichever you prefer (within your hospital's policies, of course). Surgeons have different preferences in many different areas; one of the ways we find which preference is most comfortable for us is by trying the different options. Whichever method of scrubbing you use, follow the directions precisely. Don't try to go too fast—like much of surgery, scrubbing will take practice—and don't follow the bad examples you may see that do a suboptimal scrub. You can do better for your patient.

Ideally, you'll have an opportunity to speak with the attending surgeon or residents at the scrub sink before entering the case. This is the time to get focused, to get ready for the task at hand. The more senior members of your team may ask you what you'd like to learn during this case or give you an idea of what the general approach to the surgery will be.

When you're done, enter the operating room by opening the door with your back, and stand in line to get a towel (if you used water) and your gown and gloves from the scrub tech. There's tradition at work here, too; though most of us don't even notice, some attending surgeons will expect that they'll be gowned and gloved before the other members of the team.

■ YOU'RE SCRUBBED IN. NOW WHAT?

Here's where you stand: out of my way, that's where. If I hear you breathe, if I see you twitch, you're out of my OR. Can't see anything? Well, that's too bad for you. Suction there. NO, there. NO, THERE!! Can't you see where the blood is?!? Remember before when I said speak when spoken to? Well, that is especially true right now. No I won't let you throw a stitch this case, but here is a retractor for you to hold for the next 6 hours. And no, I don't care how much your arm hurts. That pain is what learning feels like.

By now, you should know that you are a valuable member of the OR team. As such, you are not expected to just cower in the corner now that the drapes are on. This is important to know from the very beginning of the case, known as the "time-out," when the surgeon or nurse reads through a checklist to ensure that all steps have been completed so the procedure can start safely. During this time, every member of the OR team should feel empowered to speak up if anything seems amiss. This means YOU. As always, this is done to ensure that we are doing the right thing to the correct patient. If you are intimidated, give the resident standing next to you a quick nudge. However, please make sure we are aware of any issues before we start. Will we be a little ashamed that a med student caught something we didn't? Perhaps. But if it leads to better care of our patient, BELIEVE US, we will be thankful.

Once the operation has begun, this should be the fun part. Yes, it's true, we might need you to hold a retractor for a bit or suction some blood away from the operative field. We are, in fact, very appreciative for this thankless work. However, you are the one paying good money to be here, and as such you should be getting something out of it, too. If you can't see what is happening in the case, let us know. We may be able to reposition you elsewhere around the patient. Perhaps the circulating nurse can get you a step stool. Advocate for yourself, and we'll try to help the best we can.

We appreciate students who are proactive in helping during the case but it can be tricky to find a happy medium. Try to pick up on our cues to the best of your ability and always think of patient and team safety when making your moves. You may have been told to never touch the scrub tech's instrument stand. This is true. He or she has this set up in a very particular way, with sharp objects that could injure you if you try to grab at things. Always ask permission if you feel like it would help the case for you to take an instrument off the tray—for your safety and the scrub tech's sanity.

After you've toiled away, hopefully seen amazing anatomy that is a true privilege to behold, all the while taking in skillful surgical technique, it's your time to shine. It's closing time. This is a part of the case where residents are typically most comfortable and happy to give up the reins. This is where you can get your first experience practicing surgical skills on a real live human being. So, when the skin suture comes onto the field, if it looks like you are getting passed over you should speak up. There might be a rush to finish up the case and you might get accidentally (or purposefully) ignored, so make your goal of participating in the closure known; also, make sure that you've been practicing your suturing outside the OR because some attendings will only let you "play" if you have been practicing via simulation. Participating in the wound closure in the OR is how you get to hone the skills that you can't develop anywhere else. This is why the OR is so great.

■ NOW THAT THE CASE IS OVER...

We're done. Get the next one ready; page me when you're prepped.

If it's a busy day, we may have already stepped out of the room while you're closing. Ideally, even if delegating the final dressings to the rest of the team, we're still available as attendings to ensure the case has gone the way that's best for the patient, as well as to ensure that the trainees at all levels have had their experience and education furthered by being a part of the team during this case. If we did have to step out, that responsibility's not passed up; we'll try to make it up to you. We may do a "debriefing" before we're even completely done with the case, or, though less than perfect, while we're getting ready for the next one. As we've talked about above, though, please do feel that you can come to us to ask questions about the case or to clarify learning points even if we haven't taken the initiative to formally debrief.

One of the tasks traditionally delegated to the most junior surgeons in the room, the lowest-ranking resident and medical student, is assisting with transporting the patient out of the operating room. This isn't meant to be yet another thankless piece of scut, but rather a display of teamwork and a safety mechanism—if something goes amiss during transport to the recovery area or ICU, you may be the person with the most direct line of communication to the attending surgeon. Not all hospitals continue this tradition; at some, the attending always stays with the patient, while at others, the surgeon leaves the patient in the able care of the anesthesiology and nursing teams. If you are accompanying the patient, give them your full attention; now's not the time to check your social media feeds (and remember that you should never, ever Tweet about what you've just been doing).

Once the patient's safely out of the OR, there's still work to do. Residents will often be writing operative notes and placing postop orders. You're encouraged to ask them to teach you how. They're there to teach, as well, and most are thrilled to do so. Learn what tests and monitoring most postoperative patients need, how to write coherent IV fluid orders, and why some patients get antibiotics after their surgery and others don't. A huge portion of surgery takes place before and after the operating room. Don't neglect this important part of your education.

◾ FEEDBACK

Yes? Do I know you? Oh, sure, you're the med student. Yeah, good job. Keep reading.

Feedback may be the most difficult part of your surgical rotation, for both you and your attending surgeon. There are many books written on how to give and accept appropriate feedback, and while we try hard, we're not perfect. We'll try to give you feedback frequently, after each case and each presentation, but we'll admit that we get distracted and busy, too. If you're seeking areas in which you might improve—and you should be—please approach us early and often regarding things you can do better. You can even reach out to our administrative assistants to perhaps schedule one-on-one time in an office setting. An interaction with an attending that doesn't lead to obtaining meaningful feedback is a wasted learning opportunity. We as attendings can easily lose sight of this, so please seek us out.

On the other hand, don't take the comments we give as simple generics that don't really apply to you. As we noted, we're not all great at the skill, but we really do want to give you feedback that meaningful for you. A short comment may seem like a throwaway, but take it to heart. If you are getting feedback as part of a group of students and residents, always assume the constructive feedback is meant for you individually, and not someone who's doing "worse" than you are.

And we've joked about it plenty, but there are unfortunately people in academic surgery who don't demonstrate the constructive, team-oriented, Uber-teacher approach that most of us desire, that most of us understand is the best culture to manage the great responsibility of patient care. You'll work with them, and, despite the difficulties, hopefully you'll learn from them. If their feedback isn't always constructive, do what you can to separate the personality from the feedback and find the nugget of useful information within their tirades. They can't always be avoided—but they can still be educational.

Thanks for joining the team, and good luck.

Tomfoolery, Shenanigans, and Hazing in Surgery

• *Luke V. Selby, MD*

■ INTRODUCTION

Like most exclusive groups, surgery has its share of rites of passage—activities ranging from the silly and harmless to those bordering on hazing. As you will soon find out, the OR can be a stressful place, and different surgeons have different ways of relieving the tension there. While some techniques are funny, harmless, and effective, not all are. Hopefully the only thing you will need to take away from this chapter is that someone managed to use the words "tomfoolery" and "shenanigans" in a medical textbook, but unfortunately this chapter exists because tomfoolery and shenanigans aren't the only things that happen in an OR. We will try to describe, from the point of view of a current surgery resident, specific events that are likely to occur in the OR and how to respond to them.

■ HARMLESS NONSENSE

OR Scut (Mostly Isn't Scut)

Most of what occurs in an OR is clearly NOT hazing. Tasks such as retracting, "driving" the camera during laparoscopic surgery, and placing a urinary catheter are necessary components of an operation. Intraoperatively, these tasks fall to students because the surgical resident and attending are needed to perform more in-depth pieces of the operation and because table space is limited. In order to get close enough to the field you have to actually be AT the field, and everyone at the field has to contribute to the operation. Providing exposure and visualization for the attending and resident gets you exposure to the operation itself and the teaching that occurs at the table. Retracting isn't the most fun part of the operation, but it is one of the more important parts (and that is why we get so annoying about keeping the retraction JUST SO). Those of you who go into surgery will doubtlessly look back at your experience as a medical student and think "That's why they were so annoying about the retraction/camera view." Not as embarrassing as the first time you say something and realize you sound like your Mom or your Dad, but close.

We ask you to place the Foley for a similar reason: there are few other opportunities for students to learn how to do it. Having you do it gives you practice and gives us a chance to assess your technical abilities and how well you respond to technical direction. If you perform well, you'll probably find yourself doing more in the operation.

Always Cutting Sutures the Wrong Length?

Every suture you cut will be the wrong length. It just will. If the resident takes your hand and places it exactly perfectly and nothing moves a millimeter before you cut it, it will still be the wrong length. This is one of the eternal truths of surgery. The correct length for a tail (the free end of suture coming off the knot) is whatever length your attending or resident tell you it is, even if 3 seconds ago it was a different length. For some reason telling medical students they cut the suture the wrong length (spoiler alert: a fair amount of time the length is fine) has propagated across all of surgery as a fun thing to do. Why? Who knows. It isn't funny. It isn't (always) true, but it is something we do (and even though I'm now forever on record saying it is silly, I'll probably still do it).

Of course, depending on the type of suture or its location, the length of the tail you leave does matter. Monofilament sutures, like PDS, can unravel and needs a longer tail to prevent the entire knot from coming undone; braided sutures, like Vicryl, can be cut closer to the knot.

To cut:

1. Take just the end of the scissors (screw facing the sky) and place it where you think the suture should be cut. Don't past-point.
2. Ask "is this length good?" If not, put the scissors at the "right" length.
3. Rotate the scissors clockwise slightly and cut. If you're cutting directly on the knot, slide your scissors down onto the knot then rotate and cut. Please, please, PLEASE don't cut the knot. You may make a grown woman or man cry if you do.

I've Never Heard That Song Before

Most surgeons listen to music in the OR, and OR conversations often shift to musical tastes with the attending asking the student (or the resident) to name the song/artist. It is just as annoying in the OR as it is when you're driving with your significant other, but it is also a way to bond, pass the time, and make fun of students for being young and not recognizing the incredibly important bands that were popular when the attending in the room was 15 (and the student probably wasn't born yet).

■ MOSTLY HARMLESS NONSENSE

Pimping

There are, of course, some things that happen in the OR that are meant in good fun but seem to an outsider to be inappropriate. The most obvious example is pimping. As you know, or will soon discover, surgery is a fast-paced environment and a lot of what we need to know we need to know instantly. One way to assess this type of knowledge is directed questions on a topic where answers expose knowledge gaps. Done well, the resident or attending asking questions will ask progressively harder questions until the student gets something wrong and then guide the student to figuring out the answer. Done poorly, the resident or attending will publicly belittle the student about the fact that they don't know an answer. The first approach is quite helpful and a good way of teaching and assessing knowledge. The second approach doesn't further any educational goals and is not helpful. Unfortunately, not all surgeons have learned this.

Blame Anesthesia, or the Resident, or the Most Junior Person in the Room

Things break in the OR. Things fall in the OR. Things go wrong in the OR. Most of the time when an instrument falls, or the suction stops working, or a needle is dull, it isn't anyone's fault. However, depending on your local culture, you may hear people "blaming" anesthesia or the residents (or medical students) for these things, especially when it clearly isn't their fault. When done in good fun this type of kidding around can be harmless (an attending blaming a resident for dropping an instrument the attending was holding), but like many jokes it is certainly possible that this type of joking can be seen as joking by one party and not by another.

No, You Probably Didn't Contaminate the Field

For obvious reasons, maintaining the sterility of the patient and the scrub table is essential in an operating room. Though you've probably been told 5000 times not to touch any of the blue stuff, you're going to be told it again. Yes, you were at least 18 inches from the scrub table, and absent an earthquake you weren't going to stumble into the table, but you still heard "Don't touch the table." So, just don't touch the table. If you contaminated yourself, don't be embarrassed, just say "I think I touched X" and (depending on what you touched, and where) you'll either need to go re-scrub, put on a new sleeve, or get a new set of gloves. We all contaminate ourselves by accident (almost always anesthesia's fault—see above), and you'll notice residents and attendings casually asking for new gloves fairly frequently. If someone tells you that you contaminated yourself, even if you didn't, thank them for pointing it out and get sterile again. Don't argue or point out that the laws of physics make it impossible for you to have touched the IV pole 3 feet from you because this is a debate that you will lose. Actually contaminating yourself happens fairly frequently and we've all been told we need to re-scrub even when we don't.

■ NOT HARMLESS, NOT NONSENSE

Someone Woke Up on the Wrong Side of the Bed (Every Day for the Last 30 Years)

As a medical student, resident, and fellow you will work with people who are having a bad day and unfairly take it out on you. You'll also probably take out your crappy day on someone else (of course I've never done it, but I'm told it happens). While part of being an adult is dealing with people who are randomly and unfairly angry, you shouldn't have to deal with that on a daily basis or repeatedly from the same individual. If you're lucky enough to train at a place where you're not profiled for being a medical student, please skip to the next chapter and count your lucky stars that you have no idea what I'm talking about. If not, you have several options. Repeated harassment is unacceptable in any circumstance, and it is always appropriate to approach your clerkship director or dean with concerns about systemic mistreatment at a clinical site or by particular individuals. You're also allowed to let it roll off your back, move on, and promise yourself you won't mistreat an entire class of workers when you're no longer the lowest person on the totem pole. Personal attacks beyond simple rudeness should never be tolerated.

My Attending Has a Potty Mouth

People will curse in the OR. The attending may curse when the resident subconsciously sabotages them and makes them drop their own scissors. They may curse when a routine operation takes a turn for the un-routine. These things happen (and there is some evidence that people who curse are more intelligent and more articulate), but they shouldn't curse AT YOU. As with pimping to embarrass, cursing at any member of the health care team doesn't accomplish anything productive and isn't even a good way to blow off steam. Keep your cursing for the traffic on your drive to work when it is still dark out, and try to have a thick skin on this stuff as long as it's not directed at you.

We're Not Michael Jordan

The only thing that should be thrown in the OR is the wrapping for your gloves, and only when doing your best jump shot or hook shot aiming at the garbage can. Try not to miss ALL THE TIME. Don't throw anything else and don't tolerate it when you see it. Throwing of instruments is a "never" event.

■ SO NOW WHAT?

The OR is an awesome place to be, and most people who work in the OR are equally awesome. Yes, some of our colleagues are "special humans," and some of what goes on is weird to an outsider. Welcome to a profession that uses "sick" as a synonym for "dying." Hopefully this chapter is nothing other than a relaxed look at a number of things you didn't know existed. If it isn't, and you think you are actually being mistreated, please speak with your institutional leadership. And, please, please, PLEASE don't cut the knot!

Hey! That suture? You left it too long when you cut it.

Post-Op (After the OR)

Privacy—Keep It To Yourself

• *Ruth Braga, MSN, RN*

Every semester, new students arrive at a large Level I trauma center to try their hand at caring for some of the toughest patients with the assistance of an experienced preceptor. Every time, we remind them of the following:

- What you do stays here.
- What you see stays here.
- What you hear stays here.
- What you say stays here.

Each incident below is an example of individuals who innocently shared just enough information that it was considered a serious violation of privacy. In some cases, the innocent person lost their job. Anything that results in the ability to identify a patient is a problem.

- Without realizing that the patient was an uncle of her Facebook friend, a scrub technician shared her frustrations over an OR case she just finished, providing details of the diagnoses, delays, and complications experienced.
- A medical student posted a selfie on Instagram without realizing that it included the patient bed board with names and physician info on it directly behind him.
- An emergency room nurse posts a photo of the torn-apart trauma bay on Instagram, with brief details of what happened to the patient who had just been there.
- Two physicians discuss the complications of an OR case on the way to the cafeteria without realizing they were walking right in front of the patient's wife.
- A student observes a large trauma in the OR, sees details of the accident on TV that evening, and proceeds to share that they were in the room during the case and the procedure that was done.

Whether you are in the hospital hallway, trauma bay, a small clinic, or visiting the OR, the rules are the same: keep it to yourself. Privacy is a serious issue, and even if you feel you are describing something without identifiers, remember that there are only a few degrees of separation between us. You never know who may be listening, watching, reading, or part of the story that you are sharing. Questions about whether you had ill intent, if it was an honest mistake, or if you would like to defend why you posted or said something are rarely asked. The only thing you will be told is to hand over your badge and gather your things.

Here are some basic tips to help you avoid problems:

- **Do not post anything on social media.** (I admit, I will post that there are days I feel like quitting/celebrating/crying/etc. about my job, but that is it. That's what "vaguebooking" is for.)
- **If it doesn't concern you, it doesn't concern you.** Literally. Our nosy instincts tell us to find out what happened to that person or how that accident happened, but if you are not providing direct care for them, it doesn't concern you. You don't get to ask follow-up questions, and you definitely don't get to look up information on them in the medical record.
- **Close the door.** If you are going to be discussing anything with patients, co-workers, fellow students, or family members, make sure you are in a private room with the door shut. Talk about your day, give report, or ask questions behind closed doors in a place you are 100 percent certain is "safe." The walls in the elevators and the hallways have ears.
- **Get privacy screens or designate private space to review/chart patient information.** Occasionally you will have the lingering family member standing over your shoulder trying to look at a patient's chart. It's not your job to share. They can go to medical records to properly request information. You aren't being rude if you ask a patient or family member how you can help them if you are concerned they are spying/snooping, and it's okay to politely remind them that you are accessing someone's confidential information and you are sure they would want their information treated the same way.
- **Log off.** A family member trying to get onto the computer to get information after you have walked away is even worse than having them standing over your shoulder. The log-off button should be your best friend.
- **No photos, please.** The office/clinic/hallway/hospital is not the place for a photo. Collecting pictures for this book was very difficult. Even with many eyes looking over them to ensure that all faces and information had been blurred (unless otherwise consented) I am still paranoid. Physicians sometimes have to take pictures of wounds, but they should only be shared through encrypted pathways without identifying information.
- **No interviews, please.** If anyone asks you about your experience, or what you just did, do not share any details. I like to stick with "I had a great day." Boring, but safe.
- **Trash it (the right way).** Clinical notes are not meant to live in the regular trashcan. Or left in the cafeteria. Or taken home. Look around and you will most likely see a locked confidential waste container nearby. Anything that has the slightest bit of patient information should be placed in these bins where you know the information will be properly disposed of.

If you are ever unclear, ask the privacy officer, physician, nurse, or any other appropriate employee at your institution. They should all know about privacy rules even if they are not directly involved in the clinical setting.

We all know how exciting the OR will be for you, and that because of it you will be eager to share. As amazing as it is, proceed with caution—it can cost you your career before it has even started.

Keep Calm and Trust the Count

- *Cynthia Howard, RN, CNC, PhD*

You've met the players. You've been initiated into the rites of the OR, which can be one of the most rewarding places to work because of the skills required, and can be the most stressful because of the skills required. Before we deal with this tension between reward and stress, I want to share several perks to working in the OR that are seldom discussed. First, you are pretty safe from being held accountable to anything embarrassing that you might do out in public; working in the OR is sometimes like being in the Witness Protection Program because no one will recognize you with your own clothes on and without the mask and hat. Many people who work in the OR have an inside joke: "I didn't recognize you with your clothes on." Also, if you don't want to talk about work in social settings, a single episode describing body fluids, open cavities, or anything else surgical will generally discourage questions about your job in the future.

There are so many great things about being in the OR that are completely unique, and these are what help to keep the stress down to a dull roar. You hear all the time about the need for great communication skills in order to work as a team. After all, "teamwork makes the dream work," and it keeps patients safe. In the OR, almost everyone is gowned and gloved with only their eyes showing, making it hard to relate to someone you are talking to as a "normal" human. With the surgeons up to their elbows in body parts, nurses and techs running around counting, slapping instruments around, answering phones and taking messages for the docs who may be belting out the lyrics to their favorite songs, you can see why it can be hard to stay focused. Some days it's like a three-ring circus. With everyone concentrating on their particular job, yet needing to stay aware of what everyone else is doing because of the potential impact on the patient, it is important to stay alert and accountable to what is happening. Because of the tension that can come from strong personalities and the difficulty of the surgery, stress reactions are common.

The stress reaction is a primitive survival instinct. It is hardwired in the nervous system, which has not changed in 200,000 years. The stress reaction is instinctive and when triggered takes over the rational part of the brain—the cortex—driving one into a response often referred to as "lizard brain" (the primitive survival instinct). When stressed, you respond not to your thoughts but to your feelings. Stress can make you act stupid. The good news is that something as simple as conscious breathing can help you to stop the stress response in its tracks. Breathe in for a count of four, hold it for a count of four, and then exhale a count of four. Repeat. This will help you focus and re-engages your cortex so your inner lizard doesn't start running around the room shouting silly things.

The body is brilliant at maintaining homeostasis and restoring so the vital organs can function properly. However, it can come at a steep price, because chronic stress can compromise the immune system, leaving you open to a host of chronic diseases. The brain, while stimulated by one set of hormones under the stress reaction, is damaged by another set of hormones when there is too much stress. The stress reaction short-circuits the brain's ability to make good decisions. The stomach lining thins out and various GI maladies can occur. The list of potential health challenges as a result of chronic stress is long. In fact, some reports indicate as many as 90 percent of visits to the doctor are due to a stress-related symptom, and over 60 percent of all disease has its origins in the stress reaction. It is important for you to manage your stress reaction and build resilience so you can continue to enjoy the OR and not pay the price of chronic stress.

Any work in the OR means being part of a highly specialized field, and if you take care of yourself outside of work, you will be able to consistently perform well on the job. In addition, emotions are contagious, and one person's mood can influence a group of people in a good or a bad way. Do you want to have less stress in your immediate environment? Manage your emotions and model this for others. You will find that your ability to be calm helps to calm everyone around you.

Using emotional intelligence (EI) can help you to defuse stressful events in the operating room through managing your emotions. The roots of EI go back to the intelligence testing movement in the early 1900s when E. L. Thorndike, professor of educational psychology at Columbia University Teachers College, first identified the concept of social intelligence. In the 1920s and 1930s, attempts to measure the "ability to deal with people" essentially failed. For the next 50 years, behaviorists dominated the field of psychology with the focus on measuring IQ. In 1995, Daniel Goleman wrote the book *Emotional Intelligence* and introduced EI in the context of performance. Goleman demonstrated the value of EI in increasing profitability in organizations as well as predicting personal effectiveness in a more compelling way than IQ ever did.

Goleman defined the following five elements of emotional intelligence:

1. Self-Awareness. Do you know your emotions, values, and goals? Do you have an inventory of your strengths and weaknesses and know (and care about) the impact you have on others?
2. Self-Regulation. Do you control yourself emotionally? Think before you act? Characteristics of self-regulation are thoughtfulness, comfort with change, integrity, and the ability to say no.

3. Motivation. Are you able to work for the long-term gain and defer immediate gratification? Characteristics include being highly productive, embracing challenges, and focusing on what is most effective.
4. Empathy. Do you identify with and understand the wants, needs, and viewpoints of those around you?
5. Social Skills. Are you easy to talk to? Are you a team player and interested in helping others move toward their goals?

Within these dimensions are additional skill subsets that can be developed, such as assertiveness, stress tolerance, awareness, and self-regard.

EI is a cornerstone of the anti-stress superpower, resilience. On a long-term basis, resilience is what you want to cultivate to stay calm and focused in even the most chaotic settings. Evaluate yourself on the five characteristics mentioned above, develop your skills there (no one is perfect at all of them), practice breathing, and engage in a regular practice of gratitude and appreciation; each of these activities will help you to activate your resilience. When you activate your resilience, you are aware of the choices you make every day, to support great health, diet, lifestyle, and sleep, and feed your spirit.

When you are in the operating room and things get stressful, don't be a lizard by just reacting. Breathe, use your kindest words, and remember that your emotions are contagious.

A Brief Post-Op Note

• *Amalia Cochran, MD, FACS, FCCM*

The most interesting part of putting this book together has been answering the question "what is the book about?" Telling people that it's about surgery but it's not a "scientific" textbook has generally been met with great (and appropriate) curiosity. When I further clarify that it is intended as a survival guide for someone new to the operating room environment, many people confess they wish they had something like this when they started out.

When Brian Belval from McGraw-Hill first approached me, I was inspired by his goal of demystifying the OR for people who are stepping into it for the first time, or for those who are simply OR-curious. Knowing that Ruth shared my passion for this sort of thing, she was a natural choice for a co-editor and she has exceeded all of my hopes as a collaborator. Even though parts of the book development process have been challenging for us, I am thrilled about what our friends and colleagues have built with us. I offer them a humble thanks for their contributions, and I offer you, our reader, a humble thanks for wanting to read their stories.

See you in the next case. Don't forget to go meet the patient in pre-op and introduce yourself as part of the team, okay?

AC
15 January 2016
Somewhere in the skies over the southeastern US

Quick Guide—Answers to the "What Ifs of the OR".... in 100 Words or Less

• *Amalia Cochran, MD, FACS, FCCM; Ruth Braga, MSN, RN; Karen Porter, BSN, RN; and Jon Worthen, MSN, RN, CNOR*

■ WHAT SHOULD I DO IF OR WHEN I.....

1. Don't know what OR I'm in?
   - Every OR has a front desk or a schedule of some sort. Ask the individuals at the desk where your doctor is going to be and how to get to that OR.
2. Don't know who my doctor is that day?
   - If you are a medical student and you are not sure where you are supposed to be, you can ask at the front desk, but it is probably best to arrange this the night before with your resident.
3. Have a question or need help?
   - Ask. If you notice something or don't feel comfortable speaking up, turn to one of the staff members and ask them. But you are always safer speaking up. If you need help, ask the circulator or scrub technician. They will help you and keep you out of trouble. Being new to this environment is hard. Ask for help.
4. Have a latex allergy?
   - Speak up before you enter the OR/start your rotation. ORs have latex-free carts that contain latex-free products, including gloves. If you are scrubbing in, the gloves will be the most important thing to grab. If you are highly sensitive, you want to make sure that the scrub technician is wearing latex-free gloves too, so the powder from their gloves does not get on your gloves.

Many ORs are working toward becoming latex free, but definitely ask if it is a concern for you.

5. Don't know my glove size?
   - You can ask others what their size is if they have similar hands, but the best way is to just try a size and see how it fits for you. Glove size is changeable—if your fingers are being strangled, or your gloves are falling off, try the next size up or down.

6. Don't know my gown size?
   - Similar to gloves, try one on and see how it fits. If your circulator is unable to tie it up behind you, chances are that you need a bigger size. In some facilities, gowns may be one size fits all.

7. Can't get my jewelry off?
   - Use all of the strategies you can think of (and then look on YouTube for more). Your jewelry must come off in order to scrub—no exceptions.

8. Contaminate myself when I'm scrubbed in or am not sure if I contaminated something?
   - That depends…you may just need a new glove, or you may need to remove your gown and scrub in again. Always ask.
   - When in doubt, throw it out. Maybe not literally. The item may be re-usable, so ask the scrub or circulator before just tossing it. If there is ever a question about whether something is contaminated or not, assume it is not sterile. You may need to change gloves or your gown if you have touched it or it touched you.

9. Forgot to put on my eye-gear?
   - Ask the circulator if they can grab some for you. To prevent this, do the pre-scrub "double-check" to make sure you have it on before scrubbing.

10. Forgot to take off my cell phone/pager before I scrubbed in?
   - Hopefully, you have an understanding nurse and you don't mind them reaching up into your gown or back pocket to retrieve these items. Keep your arms up at all times and be careful that you don't contaminate yourself as they reach for it. It will only take one time and you won't forget again.

11. Did not tie my scrub pants tightly enough?
   - One of the worst feelings is to feel those pants sliding down, when your hands are completely powerless. Gradually spreading your legs apart to keep them up is a temporary fix, but scrubbing out to tighten them, or asking your circulator very nicely to re-tie them for you are really your only options. Avoid this by making sure your pants are tied tightly before you scrub. Double-knots can be your best friend.

12. Need to change places or move around the room?
   - Step away from the field carefully. Always face the field. If you are trading places, pass the person front-to-front or back-to-back, so that you are always aware of where the field is in relation to you.

13. Need to sneeze?
   - The instinct is to turn your face and sneeze in the elbow. In the OR, simply step back and sneeze directly into your mask. You may want to change the mask as soon as you can.

14. Have a runny nose?
    - One of the worst things is to have a cold in the OR. If possible, don't come to work. If not, placing bits of gauze or Kleenex in your nose may be helpful. Otherwise, there isn't much you can do aside from good decongestants and lots of fluids. Change your mask and wash your hands frequently.
15. Have an itch?
    - There's not much you can do here. Wait. Ignore it. Ask the circulator to scratch it for you. Use the corner of a piece of equipment to scratch against like a bear rubbing against a tree. Remember: if you are scrubbed in, your hands cannot touch anything outside of that nipple-to-navel region. As soon as they do, you are contaminated.
16. Need to adjust my glasses?
    - Ah, this one has gotten me kicked out of the sterile field before. Why? It's a habit that I don't think of. Remember the zone for your hands. Glasses aren't sterile. Ask for help and someone will re-adjust them for you. If you touch them, you are contaminated. If you are worried that you will reach up without thinking, a visit to the store for an inexpensive set of ties for your glasses is worth it. Those will ensure they stay up on your face and remind your brain to not touch them.
17. Drop an instrument or other sterile item?
    - You need a new one. If you are scrubbed in and you have been tasked with making sure the suction tube or other awkward piece of equipment doesn't fall, watch it. Anything that falls past the level of the patient/OR table is considered contaminated. If you plan on being a hero and catching it as it falls, make sure you do it *before* it gets below the level of the table.
18. Feel sick?
    - The combination of heat, smells, lights, and other fun of the OR can make everyone a little woozy on occasion. Be sure to eat breakfast and use the restroom before coming to the OR. If you feel sick, don't feel bad about telling the circulator, "I have to sit down for a minute." If you are lightheaded, sit with your head down to get as much blood flow to the brain as possible. We'd much rather have you sit down and contaminate yourself than do what comes next. These feelings hit everyone at some point so don't feel bad about speaking up.
19. Actually pass out?
    - You will get a lot of attention. Thankfully, anesthesia is right there. We try to get you to sit down before it comes to this. You may feel silly, but nothing thrills a surgeon more than having you fall face first into the open, sterile wound of his/her patient (yes, this has actually happened). Definitely a good reason to sit. Listen to your body. Step out, get a drink and some fresh air. Take a break. We'll help you back in when you are ready.
20. Need to go to the bathroom?
    - Make sure this is part of your pre-scrub routine. Hydration is very important, but you know your bladder best. If you need to go, let the resident or attending know you will be stepping out, and remove your gown and gloves. Get a new set of gown and gloves for the circulator to open for use

when you return. Wash your hands when you exit the OR and definitely after using the restroom. You'll need to repeat the full scrub process (not waterless) to come back in.

21. Am holding retractors and my hand starts tingling?

   • Let the surgeon know that your hand is going numb and ask if you can change hand positions. A critical part of the procedure could be happening at that moment and you don't want to be moving around. The surgeon will let you know when you can switch. Communication is definitely the key here. Ask before you move.

22. Am asked for the left-handed Otis Elevators or sterile Fallopian Tubes?

   • Beware the trap! A classic trick in some operating rooms, these don't exist (at least, not as items in an OR). Although these tend to get a "Ha ha, very funny" reaction, keep in mind that if something were to happen and they needed something real while you were off looking for a fictional item, this little joke just became a patient safety issue.

23. Am at the end of my shift and relief hasn't arrived yet?

   • Circulators, scrub technicians, and anesthesia personnel should never leave the room until their replacement is within hands' reach of the patient. That means physically in the room and announcing themselves as your replacement. This can result in a longer-than-planned shift. Communicate with the charge nurse or the OR front desk to let them know that no one has come. It could be just a simple oversight. Or you may be stuck until the end of the operation.

24. Am asked by a surgeon to leave one operating room and go into another?

   • This may happen—especially to a student. If you leave one OR to go to another, you must remove your gown and gloves, wash your hands, go to the other OR, give the circulator a new gown and set of gloves to open, then step out and perform a surgical scrub again. Circulators cannot cover two rooms, scrub technicians cannot stand at two fields, and anesthesia cannot control two airways. These staff must physically remain with the one patient they are assigned to until someone in their role relieves them. Anesthesia cannot stand in for the circulator (or vice versa).

If you are orienting, training, or rotating in any position in the operating room, check with your preceptor before leaving the room or stepping away from the field (unless you are about to be sick—then just go). Even if you feel your role is unimportant (it never is), the moment you leave will be the moment you are asked for something.

Index

9 781259 587283